FAVORITE BRAND NAME

DIABETIC

DESSERTS

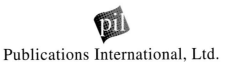

Publications International, Ltd.

Favorite Brand Name Recipes at www.fbnr.com

Nutritional Analysis: Linda R. Yoakam, M.S., R.D., L.D.

Pictured on the front cover: Lemon Raspberry Tiramisu *(page 86)*.

Pictured on the back cover *(clockwise from top left):* Holiday Thumbprint Cookies *(page 36)*, Florida Sunshine Cups *(page 8)* and Bittersweet Chocolate Torte *(page 82)*.

ISBN: 0-7853-8093-0

Manufactured in U.S.A.

8 7 6 5 4 3 2 1

Nutritional Analysis: The nutritional information that appears with each recipe was submitted in part by the participating companies and associations. Every effort has been made to check the accuracy of these numbers. However, because numerous variables account for a wide range of values for certain foods, nutritive analyses in this book should be considered approximate.

Microwave Cooking: Microwave ovens vary in wattage. Use the cooking times as guidelines and check for doneness before adding more time.

Preparation/Cooking Times: Preparation times are based on the approximate amount of time required to assemble the recipe before cooking, baking, chilling or serving. These times include preparation steps such as measuring, chopping and mixing. The fact that some preparations and cooking can be done simultaneously is taken into account. Preparation of optional ingredients and serving suggestions is not included.

table of
contents

For the Way You Live

Sacrifice no more! Crunchy cookies, decadent cakes, scrumptious cheesecakes, creamy puddings and fruity pies aren't only found in your dreams. Discover the many wonderful recipes this cookbook has to offer and enjoy the simple pleasures in life. With *Diabetic Desserts,* it's easy to make all your dessert fantasies reality.

Facts About the Recipes

The recipes in this publication were selected for people with diabetes in mind. All are based on the principles of sound nutrition as outlined by the Dietary Guidelines developed by the United States Department of Agriculture and the United States Department of Health and Human Services, making them perfect for the entire family. Although the recipes in the publication are not intended as a medically therapeutic program, nor as a substitute for medically approved meal plans for individuals with diabetes, they contain amounts of calories, fat, cholesterol, sodium and sugar that will fit easily into an individualized meal plan designed by your physician, registered dietitian and you.

The ban on sugar has been lifted for people with diabetes, but it is not altogether gone. The new guidelines for sugar intake are based on scientific research that indicates that carbohydrate in the form of sugars does not raise blood sugar levels more rapidly than other types of carbohydrate-containing food. What is more important is the total amount of carbohydrate consumed, not the source. However, keep in mind that sweets and other sugar-containing foods are often high in calories and fat and contain few, if any, other nutrients. If you have any questions or concerns about the use of sugar in your diet, consult your physician and registered dietitian for more information.

Facts About the Exchanges

The nutrition information that appears with each recipe was calculated by an independent nutrition consulting firm, and the Dietary Exchanges are based on the Exchange Lists for Meal Planning developed by the American Diabetes Association/The American Dietetic Association. Every effort has been made to check the accuracy of these numbers. However, because numerous variables account for a wide range of values in certain foods, all analyses that appear in the book should be considered approximate.

- The analysis of each recipe includes all the ingredients that are listed in that recipe, *except* ingredients labeled as "optional" or "for garnish." Nutritional analysis is provided for the primary recipe only, not for the recipe variations.

- If a range is offered for an ingredient, the *first* amount given was used to calculate the nutrition information.

- If an ingredient is presented with an option ("3 tablespoons margarine or butter," for example), the *first* item listed was used to calculate the nutrition information.

Sugar Substitutes

Every recipe in this cookbook using a sugar substitute was developed using aspartame sweetener. Before making any of these recipes, check to see what kind of sugar substitute you are using (aspartame, acesulfame-K or saccharin). Look at the package carefully and use the amount necessary to equal the granulated sugar equivalent called for in each recipe. Follow the chart below for some general measurements.

Amount of Sugar Substitute Packets to Substitute for Granulated Sugar			
Granulated Sugar	**Aspartame**	**Acesulfame-K**	**Saccharin**
2 teaspoons	1 packet	1 packet	⅛ teaspoon
1 tablespoon	1½ packets	1¼ packets	⅓ teaspoon
¼ cup	6 packets	3 packets	3 packets
⅓ cup	8 packets	4 packets	4 packets
½ cup	12 packets	6 packets	6 packets

sweet
spoonfuls

Florida Sunshine Cups

Makes 6 servings

Prep Time: 20 minutes
Refrigerate Time: 4½ hours

> ¾ cup boiling water
> 1 package (4-serving size) JELL-O® Brand Orange or Lemon
>   Flavor Sugar Free Low Calorie Gelatin
> 1 cup cold orange juice
> ½ cup fresh raspberries
> 1 can (11 ounces) mandarin orange segments, drained

STIR boiling water into gelatin in large bowl at least 2 minutes until completely dissolved. Stir in cold juice. Refrigerate 1½ hours or until thickened (spoon drawn through leaves definite impression).

MEASURE ¾ cup thickened gelatin into medium bowl; set aside. Stir fruit into remaining gelatin. Pour into serving bowl or 6 dessert dishes.

BEAT reserved gelatin with electric mixer on high speed until fluffy and about doubled in volume. Spoon over gelatin in bowl or dishes. Garnish as desired.

REFRIGERATE 3 hours or until firm.

Nutrients per serving: 1 sunshine cup
Calories: 50, Calories from Fat: 3%, Total Fat: <1g, Saturated Fat: <1g, Cholesterol: 0mg, Sodium: 46mg, Carbohydrate: 10g, Fiber: 1g, Protein: 1g

Dietary Exchanges: 1 Fruit

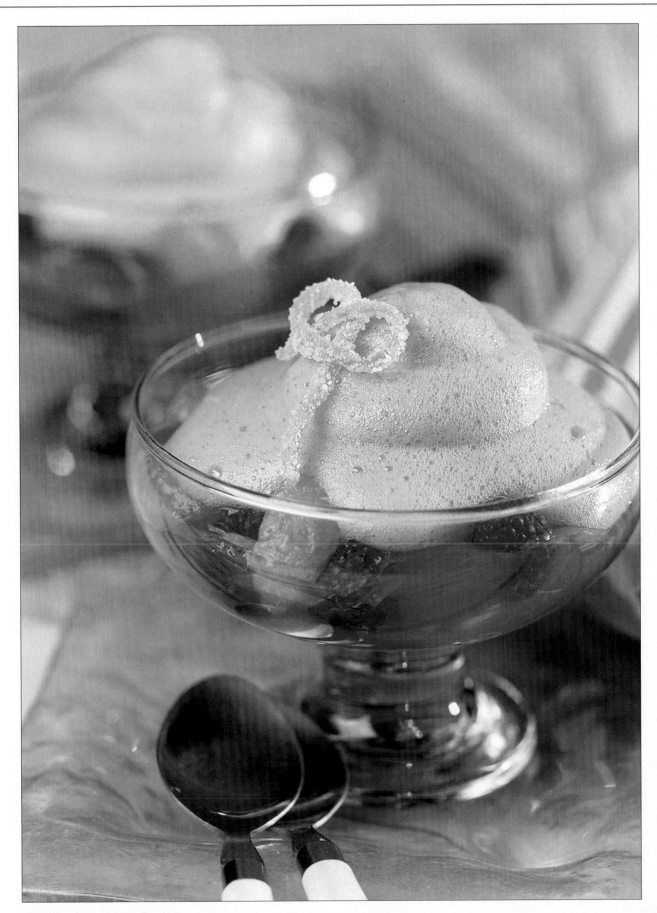

Florida Sunshine Cups

Rice Pudding Mexicana

Makes 6 servings

Prep and Cook Time: 18 minutes

> **1 package instant rice pudding**
> **1 tablespoon vanilla**
> **¼ teaspoon ground cinnamon**
> **Dash ground cloves**
> **¼ cup slivered almonds**
> **Additional ground cinnamon**

Prepare rice pudding according to package directions.

Remove pudding from heat; stir in vanilla, ¼ teaspoon cinnamon and cloves. Pour into individual dessert dishes.

Sprinkle with almonds and additional cinnamon. Serve warm.

Nutrients per serving: 1 dessert cup
Calories: 146, Calories from Fat: 27%, Total Fat: 4g, Saturated Fat: 1g, Cholesterol: 6 mg, Sodium: 106mg, Carbohydrate: 22g, Fiber: 1g, Protein: 4g

Dietary Exchanges: 1 Starch, ½ Milk, ½ Fat

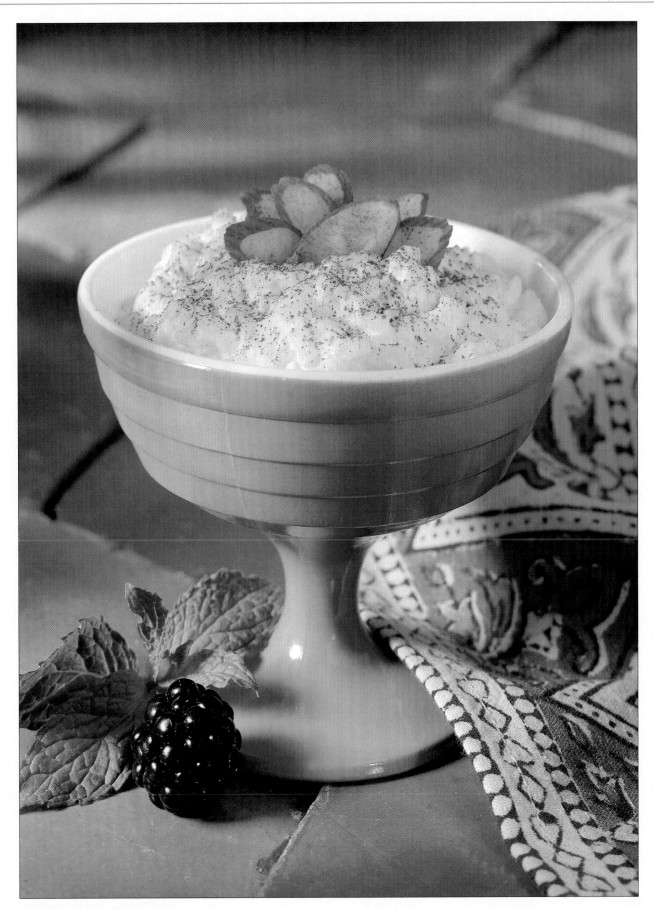

Rice Pudding Mexicana

11

Three-Melon Soup

Makes 4 servings

> 3 cups cubed seeded watermelon
> 3 tablespoons unsweetened pineapple juice
> 2 tablespoons lemon juice
> ¼ cantaloupe melon
> ⅛ honeydew melon

Combine watermelon, pineapple juice and lemon juice in blender; process until smooth. Chill at least 2 hours or overnight.

Scoop out balls of cantaloupe and honeydew.

To serve, pour watermelon mixture into shallow bowls; garnish with cantaloupe and honeydew.

Nutrients per serving: ¼ of total recipe
Calories: 68, Calories from Fat: 8%, Total Fat: 1g, Saturated Fat: <1g, Cholesterol: 0mg, Sodium: 9mg, Carbohydrate: 16g, Fiber: 1g, Protein: 1g

Dietary Exchanges: 1 Fruit

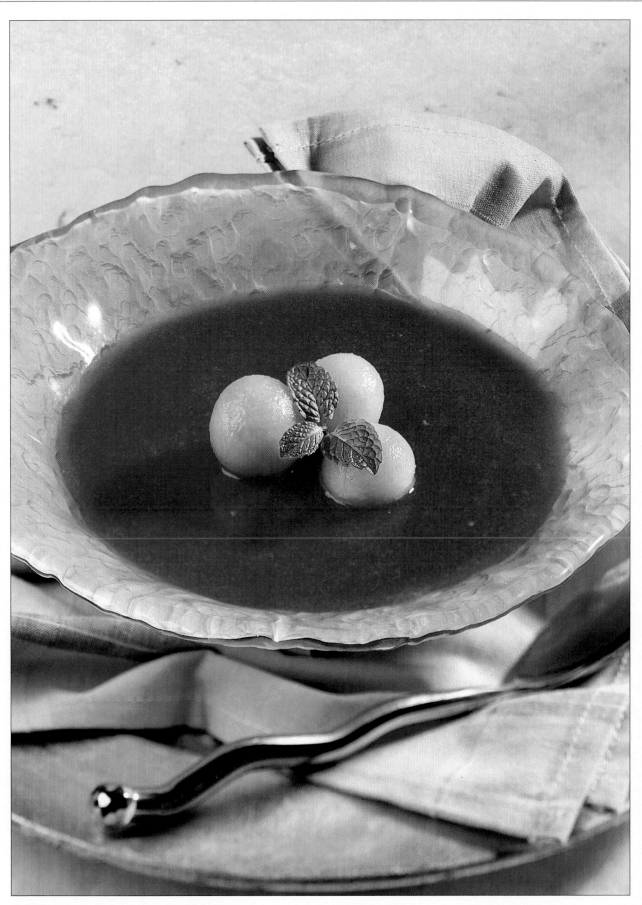

Three-Melon Soup

Refreshing Cocoa-Fruit Sherbet

Makes 8 servings

    1 ripe medium banana
1½ cups orange juice
    1 cup (½ pint) half-and-half
  ½ cup sugar
  ¼ cup HERSHEY'S Cocoa

Slice banana into blender container. Add orange juice; cover and blend until smooth. Add remaining ingredients; cover and blend well. Pour into 8- or 9-inch square pan. Cover; freeze until hard around edges.

Spoon partially frozen mixture into blender container. Cover; blend until smooth but not melted. Pour into 1-quart mold. Cover; freeze until firm. Unmold onto cold plate and slice. Garnish as desired.

Nutrients per serving: ⅛ of mold
Calories: 130, Calories from Fat: 26%, Total Fat: 4g, Saturated Fat: 2g, Cholesterol: 11mg, Sodium: 13mg, Carbohydrate: 23g, Fiber: 1g, Protein: 2g

Dietary Exchanges: 1½ Starch, ½ Fat

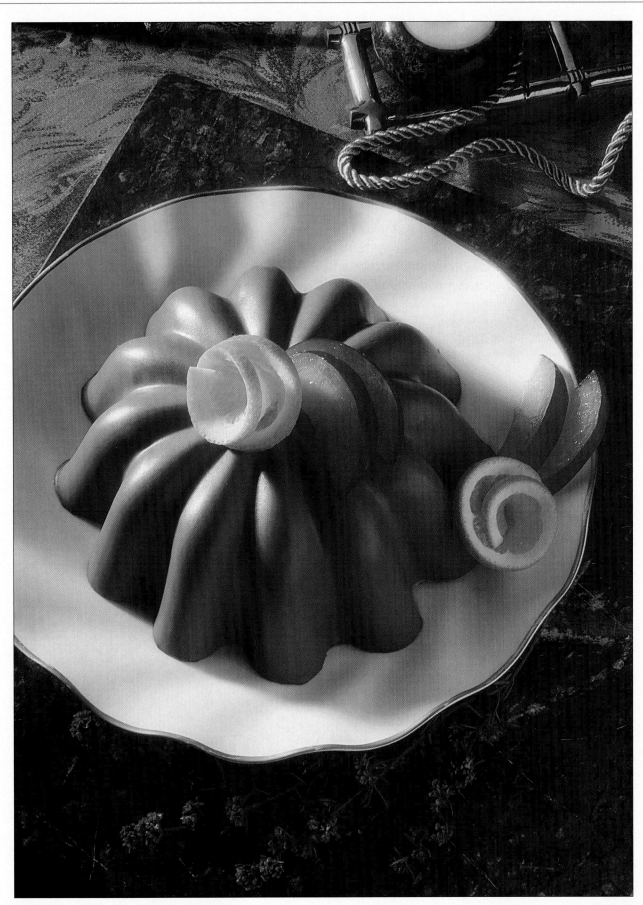

Refreshing Cocoa-Fruit Sherbet

Fresh Fruit Parfaits

Makes 6 servings

Preparation Time: 20 minutes
Refrigerating Time: 2 hours

> **1 cup fresh fruit**
> **¾ cup boiling water**
> **1 package (4-serving size) JELL-O® Brand Sugar Free Low Calorie Gelatin Dessert or JELL-O® Brand Gelatin Dessert, any flavor**
> **½ cup cold water**
> **Ice cubes**
> **¾ cup thawed COOL WHIP FREE® or COOL WHIP LITE® Whipped Topping**

DIVIDE fruit among 6 parfait glasses.

STIR boiling water into gelatin in medium bowl at least 2 minutes until completely dissolved. Mix cold water and ice cubes to make 1¼ cups. Add to gelatin, stirring until slightly thickened. Remove any remaining ice. Measure ¾ cup of the gelatin; pour into parfait glasses. Refrigerate 1 hour or until set but not firm (gelatin should stick to finger when touched and should mound).

STIR whipped topping into remaining gelatin with wire whisk until smooth. Spoon over gelatin in glasses.

REFRIGERATE 1 hour or until firm. Garnish as desired.

Nutrients per serving: 1 parfait, using ½ cup *each* blueberries and strawberries, JELL-O® Brand Sugar Free Low Calorie Gelatin Dessert and COOL WHIP FREE® (without cookies)
Calories: 46, Calories from Fat: 1%, Total Fat: <1g, Saturated Fat: <1g, Cholesterol: 0mg, Sodium: 38mg, Carbohydrate: 9g, Fiber: 1g, Protein: 1g

Dietary Exchanges: 1 Fruit

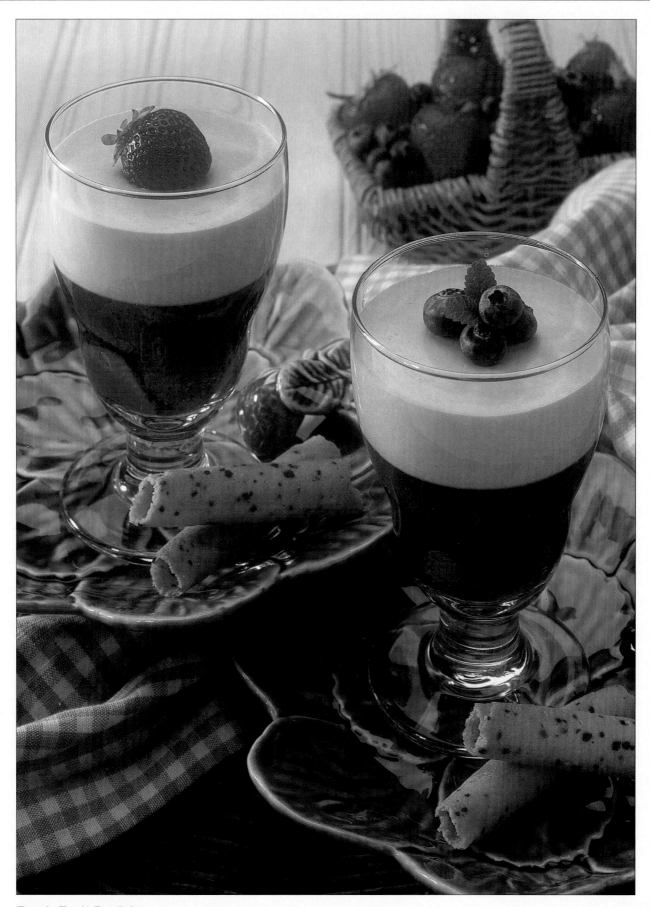

Fresh Fruit Parfaits

Yogurt Fluff

Makes 5 servings

Preparation Time: 10 minutes
Refrigerating Time: 1½ hours

> ¾ **cup boiling water**
> 1 **package (4-serving size) JELL-O® Brand Sugar Free Low
>   Calorie Gelatin Dessert or JELL-O® Brand Gelatin
>   Dessert, any flavor**
> ½ **cup cold water or fruit juice**
>   **Ice cubes**
> 1 **container (8 ounces) BREYERS® Vanilla Lowfat Yogurt**
> ½ **teaspoon vanilla (optional)**
> 5 **tablespoons thawed COOL WHIP FREE® or COOL WHIP
>   LITE® Whipped Topping**

STIR boiling water into gelatin in large bowl at least 2 minutes until completely dissolved.

MIX cold water and ice cubes to make 1 cup. Add to gelatin, stirring until slightly thickened. Remove any remaining ice. Stir in yogurt and vanilla. Pour into dessert dishes.

REFRIGERATE 1½ hours or until firm. Top with whipped topping.

Nutrients per serving: ⅕ of total recipe, using JELL-O® Brand Sugar Free Low Calorie Gelatin Dessert, water and COOL WHIP FREE®
Calories: 61, Calories from Fat: 13%, Total Fat: 1g, Saturated Fat: <1g, Cholesterol: 3mg, Sodium: 92mg, Carbohydrate: 9g, Fiber: 0g, Protein: 3g

Dietary Exchanges: 1 Starch

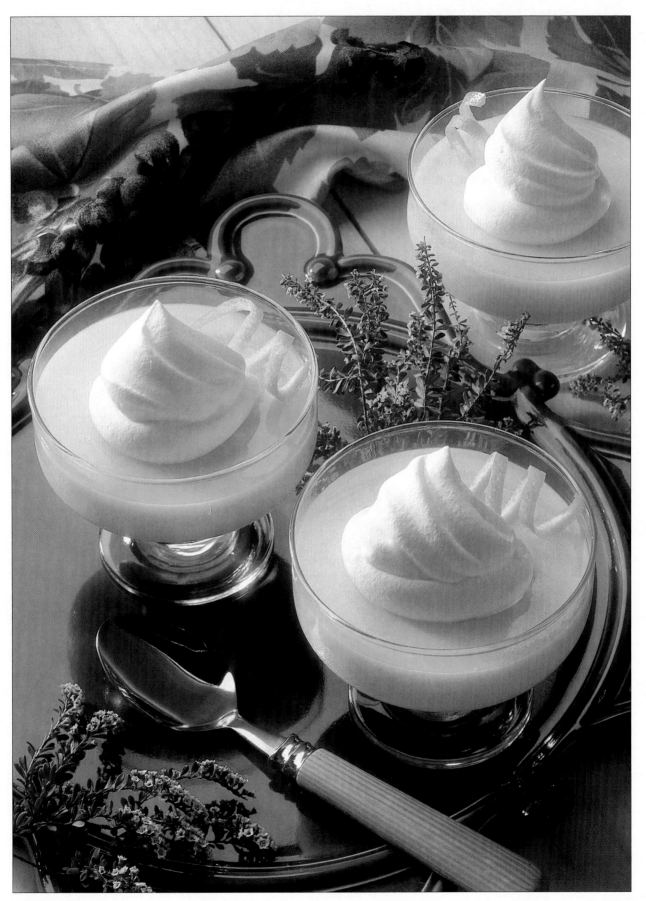

Yogurt Fluff

Peach Melba Dessert

Makes 8 servings

Preparation Time: 20 minutes
Refrigerating Time: 6 hours

> **1½ cups boiling water, divided**
> **2 packages (4-serving size each) JELL-O® Brand Raspberry Flavor Sugar Free Low Calorie Gelatin Dessert or JELL-O® Brand Raspberry Flavor Gelatin Dessert, divided**
> **1 container (8 ounces) BREYERS® Vanilla Lowfat Yogurt**
> **1 cup raspberries, divided**
> **1 can (8 ounces) peach slices in juice, undrained**
> **Cold water**

STIR ¾ cup boiling water into 1 package of gelatin in large bowl at least 2 minutes or until completely dissolved. Refrigerate about 1 hour or until slightly thickened (consistency of unbeaten egg whites). Stir in yogurt and ½ cup raspberries. Reserve remaining raspberries for garnish. Pour gelatin mixture into serving bowl. Refrigerate about 2 hours or until set but not firm (gelatin should stick to finger when touched and should mound).

MEANWHILE, drain peaches, reserving juice. Add cold water to reserved juice to make 1 cup; set aside. Stir remaining ¾ cup boiling water into remaining package gelatin in large bowl at least 2 minutes until completely dissolved. Stir in measured juice and water. Refrigerate about 1 hour or until slightly thickened (consistency of unbeaten egg whites).

RESERVE several peach slices for garnish; chop remaining peaches. Stir chopped peaches into slightly thickened gelatin. Spoon over gelatin layer in bowl. Refrigerate 3 hours or until firm. Top with reserved peach slices and raspberries.

Nutrients per serving: ⅛ of total recipe, using JELL-O® Brand Raspberry Flavor Sugar Free Low Calorie Gelatin Dessert
Calories: 64, Calories from fat: 9%, Total Fat: 1g, Saturated Fat: <1g, Cholesterol: 2mg, Sodium: 81mg, Carbohydrate: 11g, Fiber: 1g, Protein: 3g

Dietary Exchanges: 1 Starch

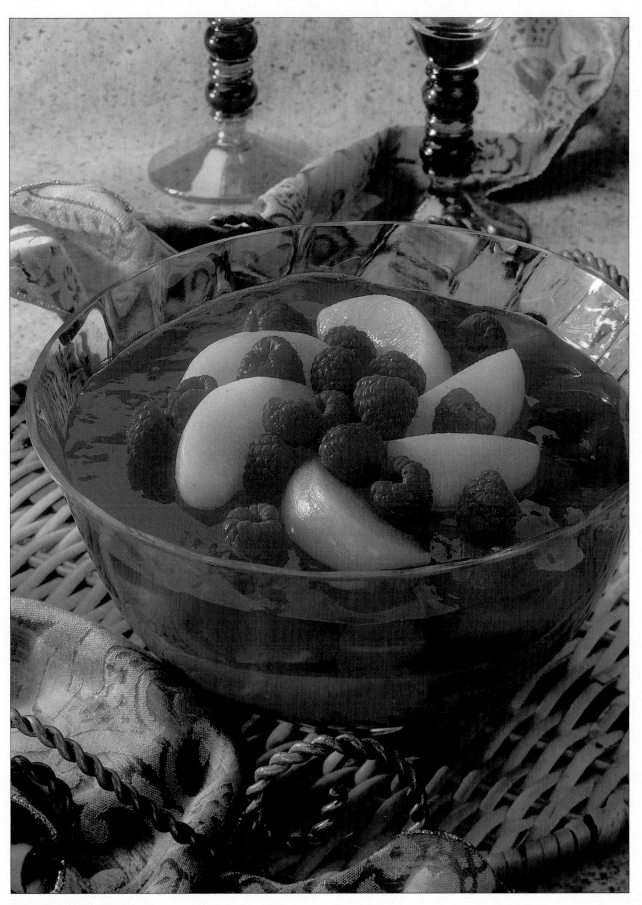

Peach Melba Dessert

Peaches & Cream Gingersnap Cups

Makes 2 servings

> 1½ tablespoons gingersnap crumbs (2 cookies)
> ¼ teaspoon ground ginger
> 2 ounces reduced-fat cream cheese, softened
> 1 container (6 ounces) peach sugar-free nonfat yogurt
> ¼ teaspoon vanilla
> ⅓ cup chopped fresh peach or drained canned peach slices
>   in juice

Combine gingersnap crumbs and ginger in small bowl; set aside.

Beat cream cheese in small bowl at medium speed of electric mixer until smooth. Add yogurt and vanilla. Beat at low speed until smooth and well blended. Stir in chopped peach.

Divide peach mixture between two 6-ounce custard cups. Cover and refrigerate 1 hour. Top each serving with half of gingersnap crumb mixture just before serving. Garnish as desired.

Note: Instead of crushing the gingersnaps, serve them whole with the peaches & cream cups.

Nutrients per serving: 1 (6-ounce) cupful dessert
Calories: 148, Calories from Fat: 34%, Total Fat: 5g, Saturated Fat: 3g, Cholesterol: 16mg, Sodium: 204mg, Carbohydrate: 18g, Fiber: 1g, Protein: 6g

Dietary Exchanges: 1 Starch, ½ Milk, 1 Fat

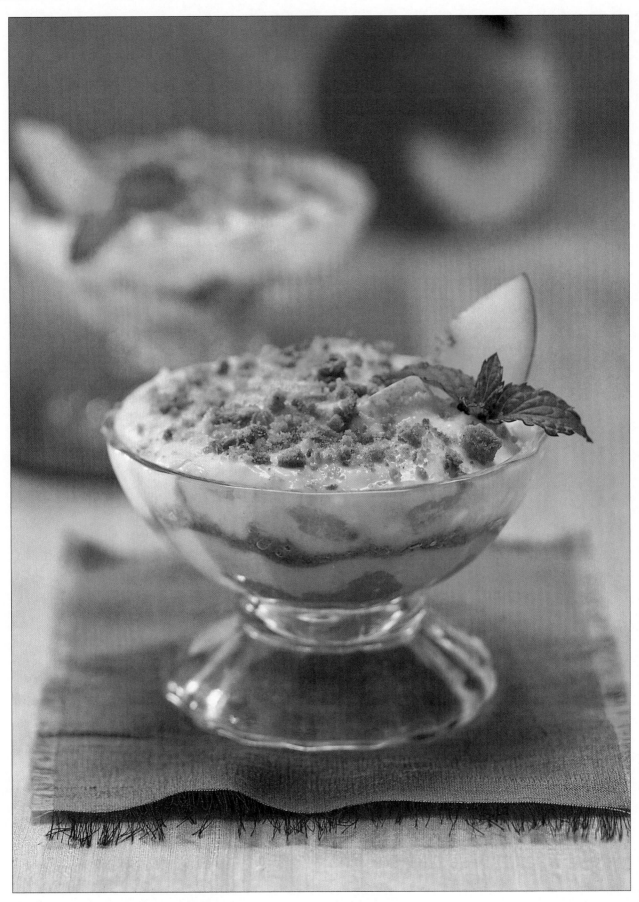

Peaches & Cream Gingersnap Cups

Peanut Butter and Jam Parfait

Makes 4 servings

Prep Time: 10 minutes

> **2 cups cold fat free milk**
> **1 package (4-serving size) JELL-O® Vanilla Flavor Fat Free
>   Sugar Free Instant Reduced Calorie Pudding & Pie Filling**
> **3 tablespoons peanut butter**
> **½ teaspoon water**
> **¼ cup fruit juice sweetened raspberry preserves**

POUR cold milk into large bowl. Add pudding mix. Beat with wire whisk 1 minute until smooth. Add peanut butter and continue beating with whisk until completely incorporated.

STIR water into preserves. Spoon about ¼ cup pudding mixture into each of 4 dessert glasses. Top with ½ of the preserves. Repeat layers. Top with additional preserves, if desired.

REFRIGERATE until ready to serve. Store leftover dessert in refrigerator.

Nutrients per serving: 1 parfait
Calories: 180, Calories from Fat: 30%, Total Fat: 6g, Saturated Fat: 2g, Cholesterol: <5mg, Sodium: 460mg, Carbohydrate: 27g, Fiber: <1g, Protein: 7g

Dietary Exchanges: 2 Starch, 1 Fat

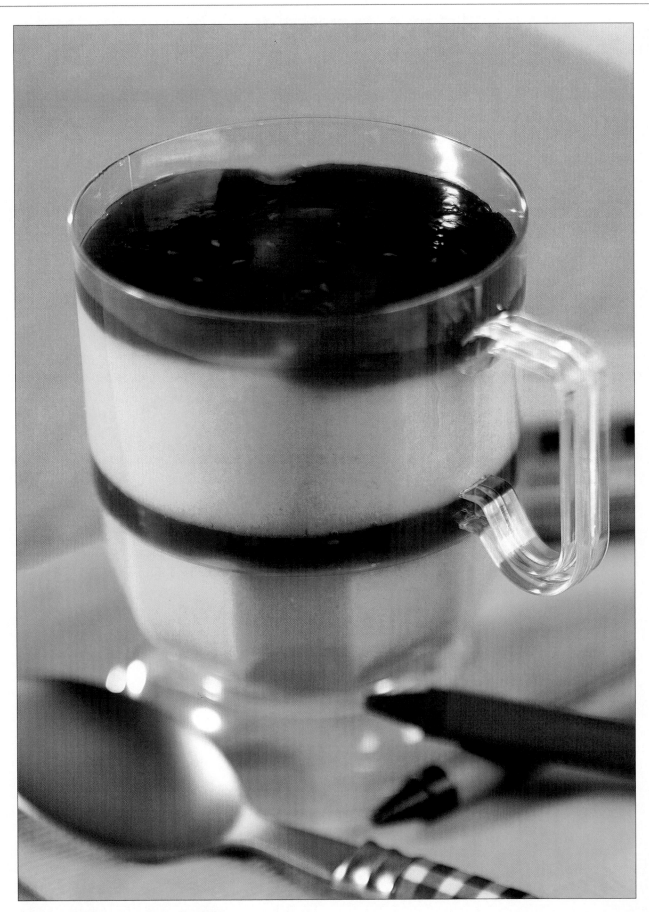

Peanut Butter and Jam Parfait

Frozen Fruit Cups

Makes 12 servings

> 1 package (8 ounces) fat-free cream cheese
> 1 cup fat-free sour cream
> 2½ teaspoons EQUAL® FOR RECIPES *or* 8 packets EQUAL®
>   sweetener *or* ⅓ cup EQUAL® SPOONFUL™
> 2 to 3 teaspoons lemon juice
> 1 cup coarsely chopped fresh *or* canned peaches
> 1 cup fresh *or* frozen blueberries
> 1 cup fresh *or* unsweetened frozen raspberries *or* halved or
>   quartered strawberries
> 1 cup cubed fresh *or* canned pineapple in juice
> 1 can (11 ounces) Mandarin orange segments, drained
> 12 pecan halves, optional

Beat cream cheese, sour cream, EQUAL® and lemon juice in medium bowl until smooth; gently mix in fruit.

Spoon mixture into 12 paper-lined muffin cups, or spread in 10×6-inch baking dish. Garnish with pecan halves and additional fruit, if desired. Freeze until firm, 6 to 8 hours.

Let stand at room temperature until slightly softened, 10 to 15 minutes, before serving.

Tip: If made in a 10×6-inch baking dish, cut into squares and serve on lettuce-lined plates as a salad or on plates with puréed strawberry or raspberry sauce for dessert.

Hint: The fruit mixture can be spooned into hollowed-out orange halves and frozen. Cut thin slices from bottoms of oranges so they will stand; place in muffin tins to freeze.

Nutrients per serving: 1 fruit cup
Calories: 81, Calories from Fat: 5%, Total Fat: <1g, Saturated Fat: <1g, Cholesterol: 2mg, Sodium: 122mg, Carbohydrate: 15g, Fiber: 2g, Protein: 5g

Dietary Exchanges: 1 Fruit, ½ Meat

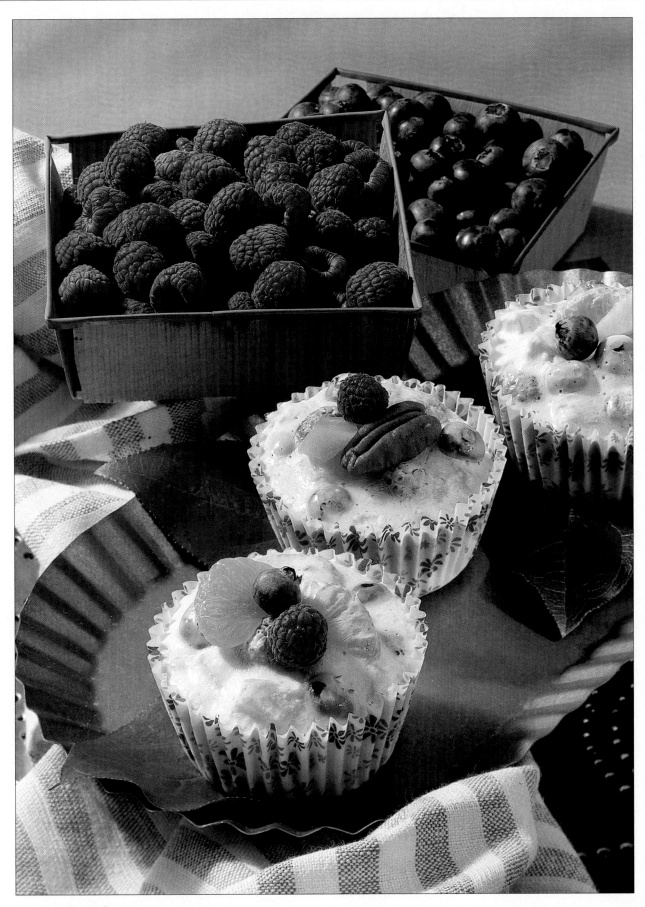

Frozen Fruit Cups

Chocolate Mousse

Makes 8 servings

- ½ **cup plus 2 tablespoons sugar, divided**
- ¼ **cup unsweetened cocoa powder**
- 1 **envelope unflavored gelatin**
- 2 **tablespoons coffee-flavored liqueur**
- 2 **cups fat-free (skim) milk**
- ¼ **cup cholesterol-free egg substitute**
- 2 **egg whites**
- ⅛ **teaspoon cream of tartar**
- ½ **cup thawed frozen reduced-fat nondairy whipped topping**

Combine ½ cup sugar, cocoa and gelatin in medium saucepan. Add coffee-flavored liqueur; let stand 2 minutes. Add milk; heat over medium heat. Stir until sugar and gelatin are dissolved. Stir in egg substitute. Set aside.

Beat egg whites in medium bowl with electric mixer until foamy; add cream of tartar. Beat until soft peaks form. Gradually beat in remaining 2 tablespoons sugar; continue beating until stiff peaks form.

Gently fold egg whites into cocoa mixture. Fold in whipped topping. Divide evenly between 8 dessert dishes. Refrigerate until thickened. Garnish as desired.

Nutrients per serving: ⅛ of total recipe
Calories: 125, Calories from Fat: 6%, Total Fat: 1g, Saturated Fat: <1g, Cholesterol: 1mg, Sodium: 60mg, Carbohydrate: 23g, Fiber: <1g, Protein: 5g

Dietary Exchanges: 1½ Starch

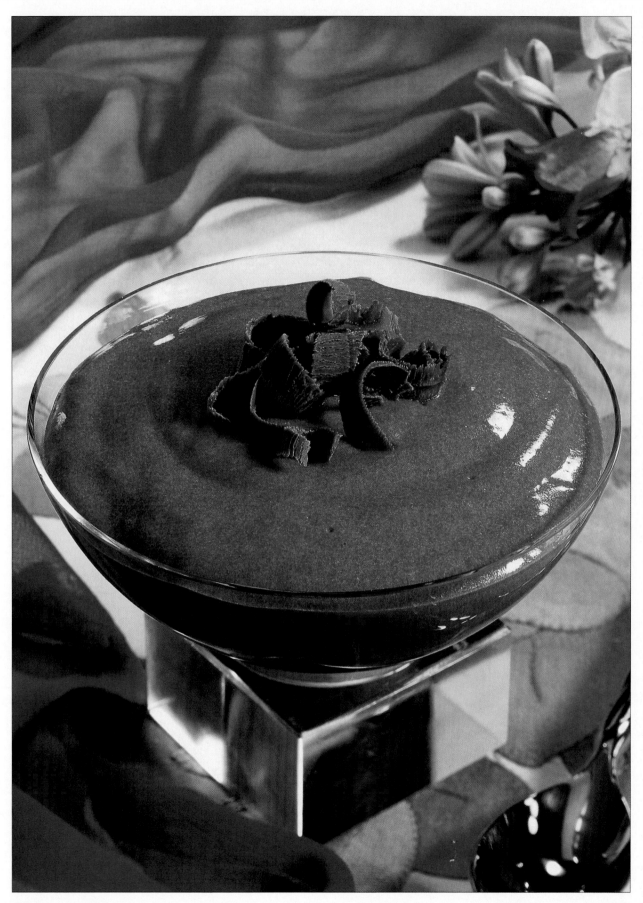

Chocolate Mousse

Paradise Parfaits

Makes 6 servings

Prep Time: 10 minutes

¼ **cup GENERAL FOODS INTERNATIONAL COFFEES® Fat Free Sugar Free French Vanilla Café Flavor**
1 **tablespoon hot water**
2 **cups cold fat free milk**
1 **package (4-serving size) JELL-O® Vanilla Flavor Fat Free Sugar Free Instant Reduced Calorie Pudding & Pie Filling**
1 **cup thawed COOL WHIP FREE® Fat Free Whipped Topping**
1½ **cups assorted fresh fruit, such as sliced strawberries, raspberries, chopped peaches *or* crushed pineapple**

DISSOLVE flavored instant coffee in hot water in medium bowl. Pour milk into coffee mixture. Add pudding mix. Beat with wire whisk 2 minutes. Gently stir in whipped topping.

SPOON ½ of the pudding mixture into 6 dessert glasses. Layer with fruit. Spoon remaining pudding mixture over fruit.

REFRIGERATE until ready to serve. Garnish with additional whipped topping and fruit, if desired.

Nutrients per serving: 1 parfait
Calories: 87, Calories from Fat: 3%, Total Fat: <1g, Saturated Fat: <1g, Cholesterol: 2mg, Sodium: 291mg, Carbohydrate: 17g, Fiber: 1g, Protein: 3g

Dietary Exchanges: 1 Starch

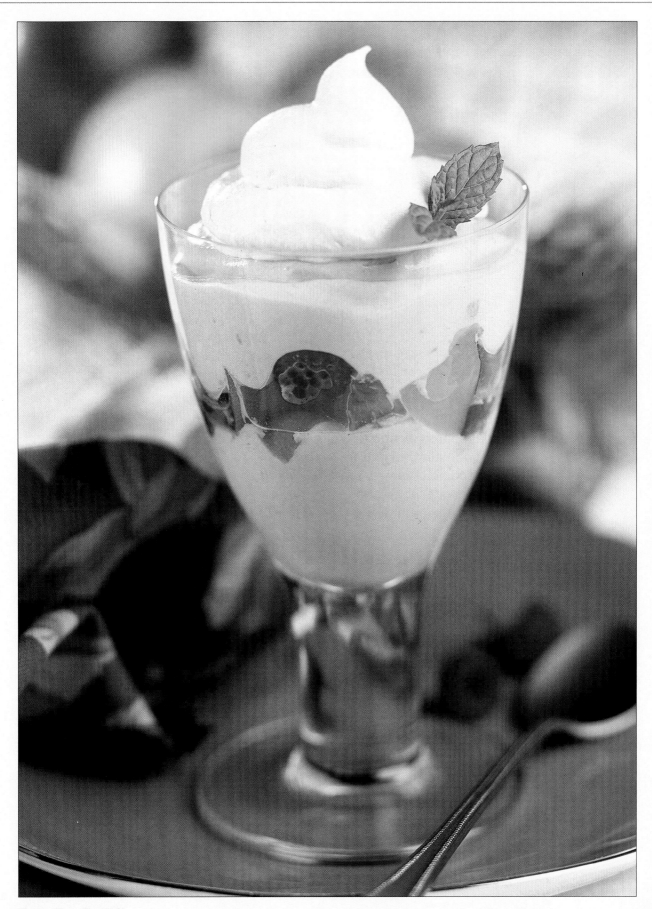

Paradise Parfait

bars &
cookies

Chocolate Cherry Cookies

Makes 20 cookies

 1 package (8 ounces) sugar-free low-fat chocolate cake mix
 3 tablespoons fat-free (skim) milk
 ½ teaspoon almond extract
 10 maraschino cherries, rinsed, drained and cut into halves
 2 tablespoons white chocolate chips
 ½ teaspoon vegetable oil

Preheat oven to 350°F. Spray baking sheets with nonstick cooking spray; set aside.

Beat cake mix, milk and almond extract in medium bowl with electric mixer at low speed. Increase speed to medium when mixture looks crumbly; beat 2 minutes or until smooth dough forms. (Dough will be very sticky.)

Coat hands with cooking spray. Shape dough into 1-inch balls. Place balls 2½ inches apart on prepared baking sheets. Flatten each ball slightly. Place cherry half in center of each cookie.

Bake 8 to 9 minutes or until cookies lose their shininess and tops begin to crack. *Do not overbake.* Remove to wire racks; cool completely.

Heat white chocolate chips and oil in small saucepan over very low heat until chips melt. Drizzle cookies with melted chips. Allow drizzle to set before serving.

Nutrients per serving: 1 cookie
Calories: 54, Calories from Fat: 18%, Total Fat: 1g, Saturated Fat: <1g, Cholesterol: 0mg, Sodium: 9mg, Carbohydrate: 12g, Fiber: 0g, Protein: 1g

Dietary Exchanges: 1 Starch

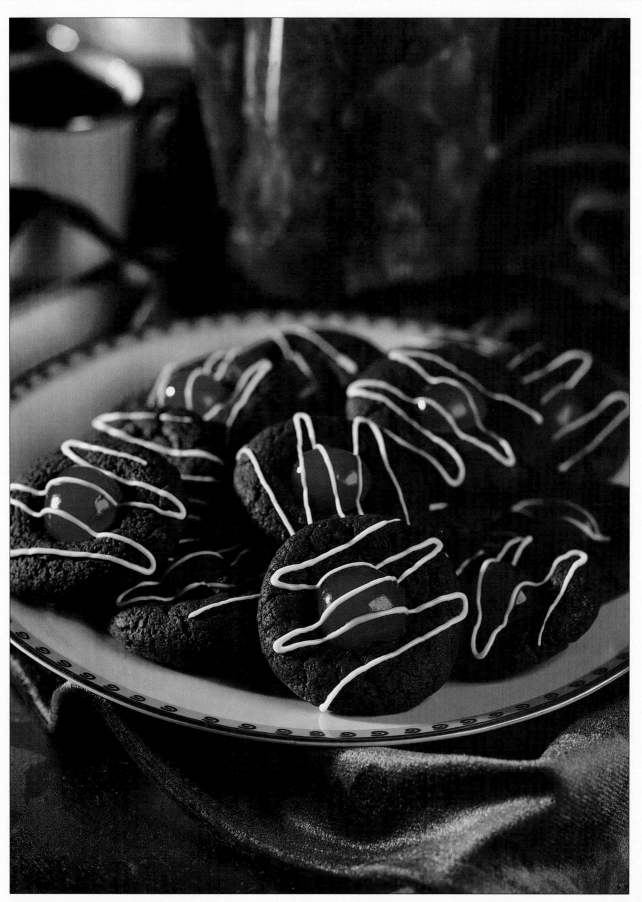

Chocolate Cherry Cookies

Hazelnut Biscotti

Makes 16 servings

> **6 raw hazelnuts**
> **2 tablespoons margarine**
> **¼ cup sugar**
> **2 egg whites, lightly beaten**
> **1½ teaspoons vanilla**
> **1½ cups all-purpose flour**
> **½ teaspoon baking powder**
> **½ teaspoon grated orange peel**
> **⅛ teaspoon salt**

Preheat oven to 375°F. Place hazelnuts in shallow baking pan; toast 7 to 8 minutes or until rich golden brown. Set aside. *Reduce oven temperature to 325°F.* Spray cookie sheet with nonstick cooking spray; set aside.

Combine margarine and sugar in medium bowl; mix well. Add egg whites and vanilla; mix well. Combine flour, baking powder, orange peel and salt in large bowl; mix well. Finely chop toasted hazelnuts; stir into flour mixture. Add egg white mixture to flour mixture; blend well.

Divide dough in half. Shape half of dough into log on lightly floured surface. (Dough will be fairly soft.) Transfer to prepared cookie sheet. Repeat with remaining half of dough to form second log. Bake both logs 25 minutes or until wooden pick inserted in center of logs comes out clean. Cool on wire racks. *Reduce oven temperature to 300°F.*

When cool enough to handle, cut each log into 8 (½-inch) slices. Place cut sides up on cookie sheets. Bake slices 12 minutes. Turn slices over; bake additional 12 minutes or until golden brown on both sides.

Nutrients per serving: 1 cookie
Calories: 76, Calories from Fat: 25%, Total Fat: 2g, Saturated Fat: <1g, Cholesterol: 0mg, Sodium: 50mg, Carbohydrate: 12g, Fiber: <1g, Protein: 2g

Dietary Exchanges: 1 Starch, ½ Fat

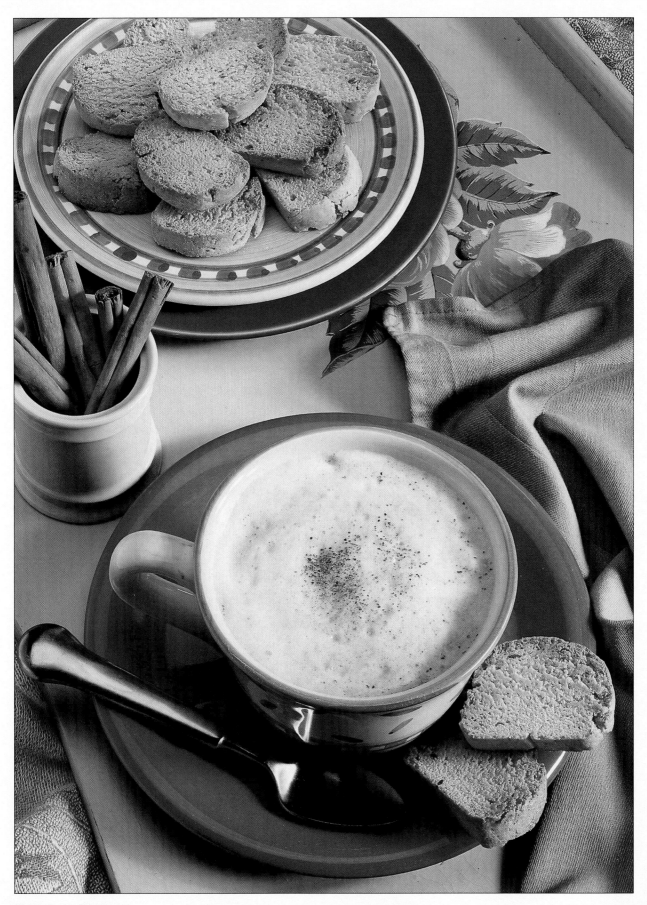

Hazelnut Biscotti

Holiday Thumbprint Cookies

Makes 20 cookies

> **1 package (8 ounces) sugar-free low-fat yellow cake mix**
> **3 tablespoons orange juice**
> **2 teaspoons grated orange peel**
> **½ teaspoon vanilla**
> **5 teaspoons strawberry all-fruit spread**
> **2 tablespoons chopped pecans**

Preheat oven to 350°F. Spray baking sheets with nonstick cooking spray.

Beat cake mix, orange juice, orange peel and vanilla in medium bowl with electric mixer at medium speed 2 minutes or until mixture looks crumbly. Increase speed to medium and beat 2 minutes or until smooth dough forms. Dough will be very sticky.

Coat hands with nonstick cooking spray. Roll dough into 1-inch balls. Place balls 2½ inches apart on prepared baking sheets. Press center of each ball with thumb. Fill each thumbprint with ¼ teaspoon fruit spread. Sprinkle with nuts.

Bake 8 to 9 minutes or until cookies are light golden brown and lose their shininess. *Do not overbake.* Remove to wire racks; cool completely.

Nutrients per serving: 1 cookie
Calories: 50, Calories from Fat: 20%, Total Fat: 1g, Saturated Fat: 0g, Cholesterol: 0mg, Sodium: 8mg, Carbohydrate: 10g, Fiber: 0g, Protein: 1g

Dietary Exchanges: ½ Starch

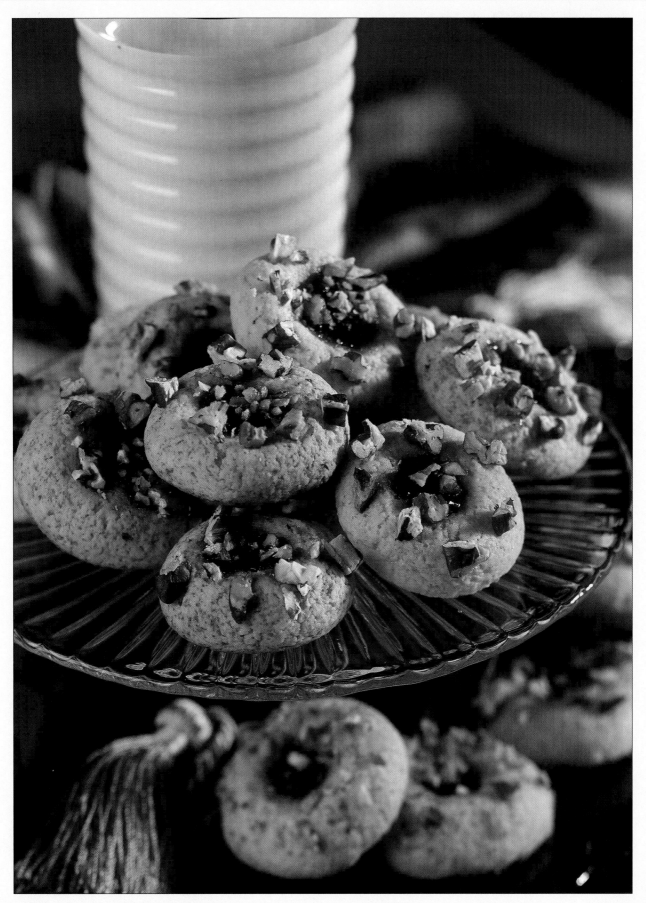

Holiday Thumbprint Cookies

Lemon Squares

Makes 16 servings

> **2 eggs**
> **5½ teaspoons EQUAL® FOR RECIPES *or* 18 packets EQUAL®**
>   **sweetener *or* ¾ cup EQUAL® SPOONFUL™**
> **¼ cup plus 2 tablespoons lemon juice**
> **4 tablespoons margarine, melted and cooled**
> **1 tablespoon grated lemon peel**
>   **Rich Pastry (recipe follows)**

Beat eggs and Equal®; mix in lemon juice, margarine and lemon peel. Pour mixture into baked pastry.

Bake in preheated 350°F oven until lemon filling is set, about 15 minutes. Cool on wire rack.

Rich Pastry

> **¾ cup all-purpose flour**
> **2½ teaspoons EQUAL® FOR RECIPES *or* 8 packets EQUAL®**
>   **sweetener *or* ⅓ cup EQUAL® SPOONFUL™**
> **2¼ teaspoons cornstarch**
> **⅛ teaspoon salt**
> **6 tablespoons cold margarine, cut into pieces**
> **1 teaspoon grated lemon peel**
> **¾ teaspoon vanilla**

Combine flour, Equal®, cornstarch and salt in medium bowl; cut in margarine with pastry blender until mixture resembles coarse crumbs. Sprinkle with lemon peel and vanilla; mix with hands to form dough.

Press dough evenly onto bottom and ¼ inch up sides of 8-inch square baking pan. Bake in preheated 350°F oven until lightly browned, about 10 minutes. Cool on wire rack.

Nutrients per serving: $1/16$ of total recipe
Calories: 104, Calories from Fat: 69%, Total Fat: 8g, Saturated Fat: 0g, Cholesterol: 27mg, Sodium: 109mg, Carbohydrate: 7g, Fiber: 0g, Protein: 1g

Dietary Exchanges: ½ Starch, 1½ Fat

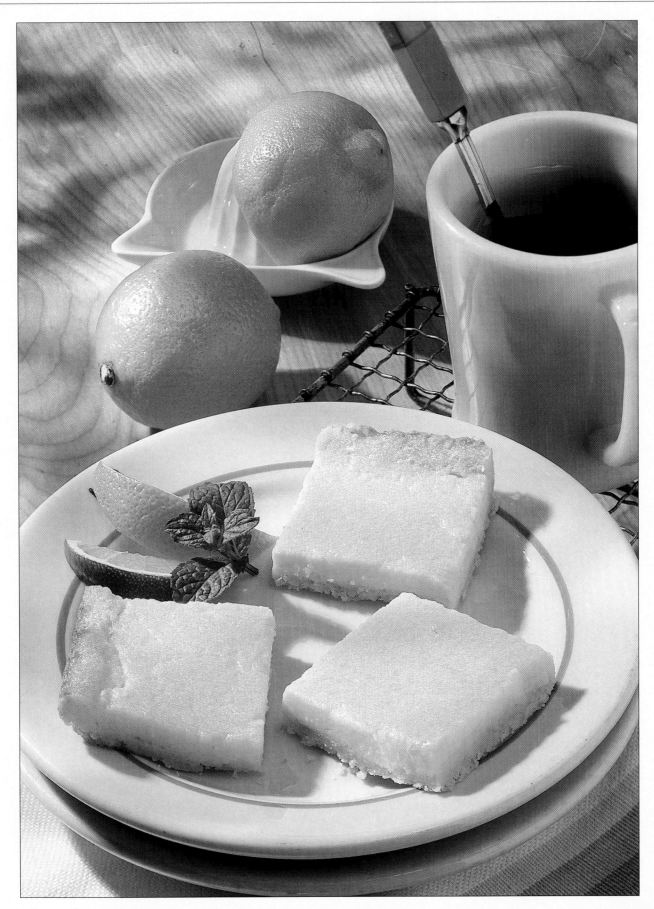

Lemon Squares

Fudgy Brownies

Makes 16 servings

> 6 tablespoons margarine
> 4 ounces unsweetened chocolate
> ⅓ cup skim milk
> ⅓ cup apricot preserves with NutraSweet® brand sweetener
>   or apricot spreadable fruit
> 1 egg yolk
> 1 teaspoon vanilla
> ½ cup all-purpose flour
> 10¾ teaspoons EQUAL® FOR RECIPES *or* 36 packets EQUAL®
>   sweetener *or* 1½ cups EQUAL® SPOONFUL™
> ½ teaspoon baking powder
> ⅛ teaspoon salt
> 3 egg whites
> ⅛ teaspoon cream of tartar
> ⅓ cup coarsely chopped walnuts (optional)

Heat margarine, chocolate, milk and apricot preserves in small saucepan, whisking frequently, until chocolate is almost melted. Remove from heat; whisk until chocolate is melted. Whisk in egg yolk and vanilla; mix in combined flour, Equal®, baking powder and salt until smooth.

Beat egg whites and cream of tartar to stiff peaks in large bowl. Fold chocolate mixture into egg whites. Fold in walnuts, if desired. Pour batter into greased 8-inch square baking pan.

Bake in preheated 350°F oven until brownies are firm to touch and toothpick inserted in center comes out clean, 18 to 20 minutes (do not overbake). Cool on wire rack. Serve warm or at room temperature.

Nutrients per serving: 1/16 of total recipe
Calories: 115, Calories from Fat: 62%, Total Fat: 9g, Saturated Fat: 3g, Cholesterol: 13mg, Sodium: 98mg, Carbohydrate: 10g, Fiber: 1g, Protein: 2g

Dietary Exchanges: ½ Starch, 1½ Fat

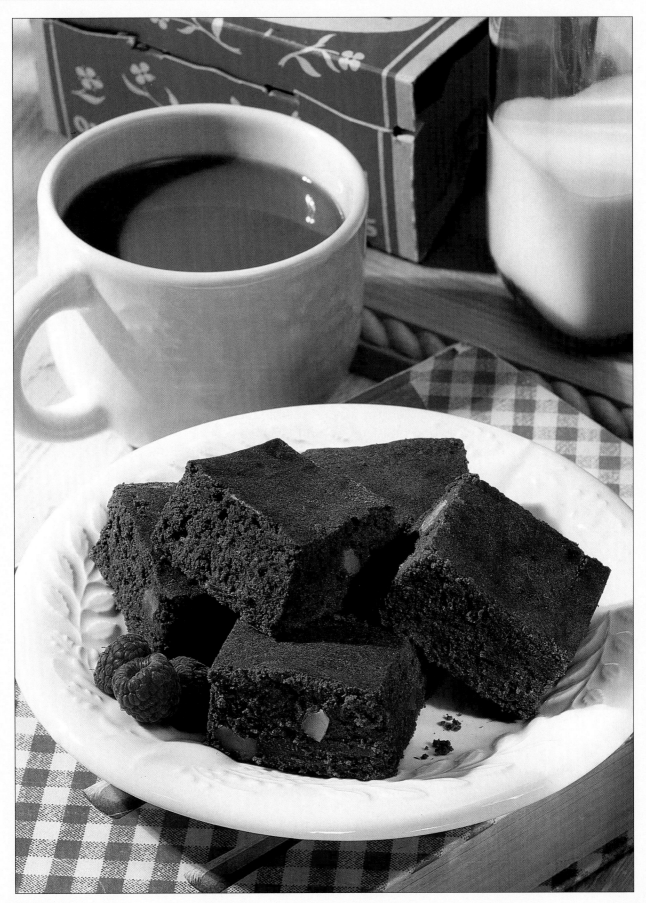

Fudgy Brownies

cakes &
cheesecakes

Brownie Cake Delight

Makes 20 servings

   1 package reduced-fat fudge brownie mix
   ⅓ cup strawberry all-fruit spread
   2 cups thawed frozen reduced-fat nondairy whipped topping
   ¼ teaspoon almond extract
   2 cups strawberries, stems removed, halved
   ¼ cup chocolate sauce

Prepare brownies according to package directions, substituting 11×7-inch baking pan. Cool completely in pan.

Whisk fruit spread in small bowl until smooth.

Combine whipped topping and almond extract in medium bowl.

Cut brownie horizontally in half. Place half of brownie on serving dish. Spread with fruit spread and 1 cup whipped topping. Place second half of brownie, cut side down, over bottom layer. Spread with remaining whipped topping. Arrange strawberries on whipped topping. Drizzle chocolate sauce over cake before serving. Garnish with fresh mint, if desired.

Nutrients per serving: ¹⁄₂₀ of dessert
Calories: 154, Calories from Fat: 14%, Total Fat: 2g, Saturated Fat: <1g, Cholesterol: <1mg, Sodium: 112mg, Carbohydrate: 33g, Fiber: <1g, Protein: 2g

Dietary Exchanges: 1½ Starch, ½ Fruit, ½ Fat

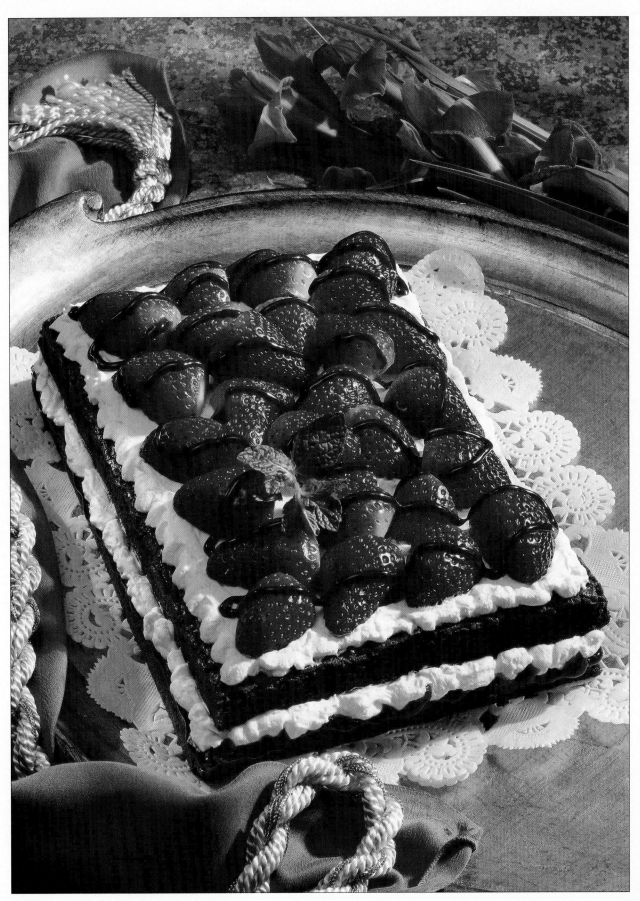

Brownie Cake Delight

German Apple Cake

Makes 10 servings

¼ cup margarine, softened
2 tablespoons strawberry spreadable fruit
5 teaspoons EQUAL® FOR RECIPES *or* 16 packets EQUAL®
    sweetener *or* ⅔ cup EQUAL® SPOONFUL™
1 egg, beaten
¼ cup skim milk
1 teaspoon vanilla
1 cup self-rising flour
1 medium Granny Smith apple
2 teaspoons lemon juice
½ teaspoon ground cinnamon
¼ teaspoon EQUAL® FOR RECIPES *or* 1 packet EQUAL®
    sweetener *or* 2 teaspoons EQUAL® SPOONFUL™

Beat margarine, spreadable fruit and 5 teaspoons Equal® for Recipes until creamy.

Blend egg, milk and vanilla; add to margarine mixture alternately with flour. (Mixture will be thick.) Spoon batter into greased and waxed-paper-lined 8-inch round cake pan.

Peel and core apple and cut into slices; toss with lemon juice. Arrange decoratively over cake batter.

Bake in preheated 350°F oven until toothpick comes out clean, about 30 minutes. Turn onto wire rack, with apple on top. Sprinkle with cinnamon and ¼ teaspoon Equal® for Recipes while cake is still warm.

Nutrients per serving: ¹⁄₁₀ of cake
Calories: 119, Calories from Fat: 40%, Total Fat: 5g, Saturated Fat: 1g, Cholesterol: 21mg, Sodium: 221mg, Carbohydrate: 16g, Fiber: 1g, Protein: 2g

Dietary Exchanges: 1 Starch, 1 Fat

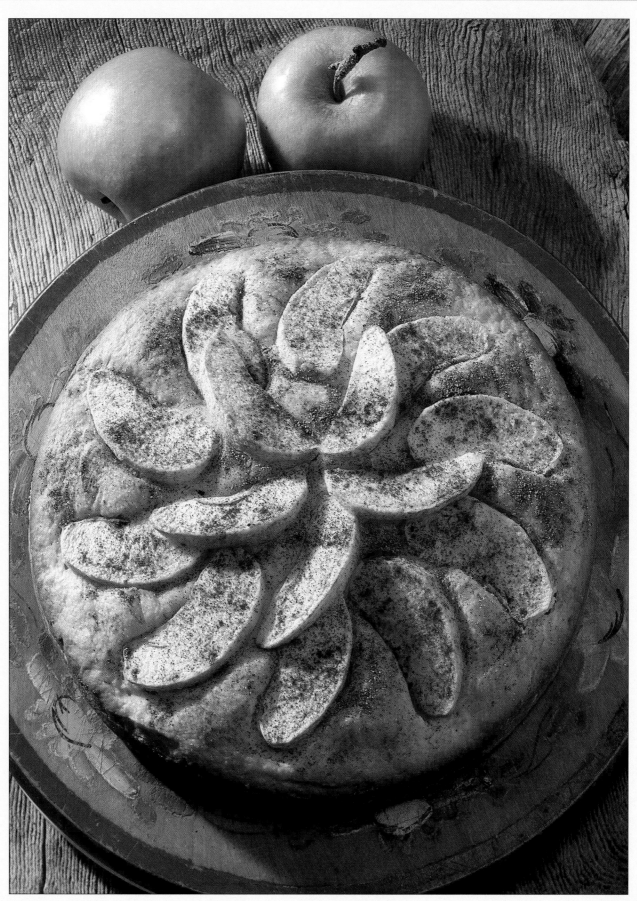

German Apple Cake

Blueberry Lemon Pudding Cake

Makes 6 servings

¼ **cup sugar**
¼ **cup all-purpose flour**
1 **cup fat-free (skim) milk**
1 **egg yolk**
3 **tablespoons fresh lemon juice**
2 **tablespoons margarine**
2 **teaspoons finely grated lemon peel**
3 **egg whites**
1 **cup sugar-free strawberry fruit spread**
2 **cups fresh or frozen (not thawed) blueberries**

Preheat oven to 350°F. Lightly spray 8-inch square glass or ceramic baking dish with nonstick cooking spray.

Combine sugar and flour in small bowl.

Combine milk, egg yolk, lemon juice, margarine and lemon peel in large bowl. Add sugar mixture to milk mixture; stir until just blended.

Beat egg whites in medium bowl until stiff, but not dry. Gently fold beaten egg whites into milk mixture; spread into bottom of prepared baking dish. Place dish in 13×9-inch baking pan; pour 1 inch hot water into outer pan. Bake 15 minutes.

Meanwhile, melt fruit spread. Drop blueberries evenly over top of cake; carefully brush with fruit spread. Bake about 35 minutes or until set and lightly golden.

Let cool slightly; serve warm or chilled.

Nutrients per serving: ⅙ of cake
Calories: 147, Calories from Fat: 29%, Total Fat: 5g, Saturated Fat: 1g, Cholesterol: 36mg, Sodium: 97mg, Carbohydrate: 22g, Fiber: 2g, Protein: 5g

Dietary Exchanges: 1 Starch, 1½ Fruit, 1 Fat

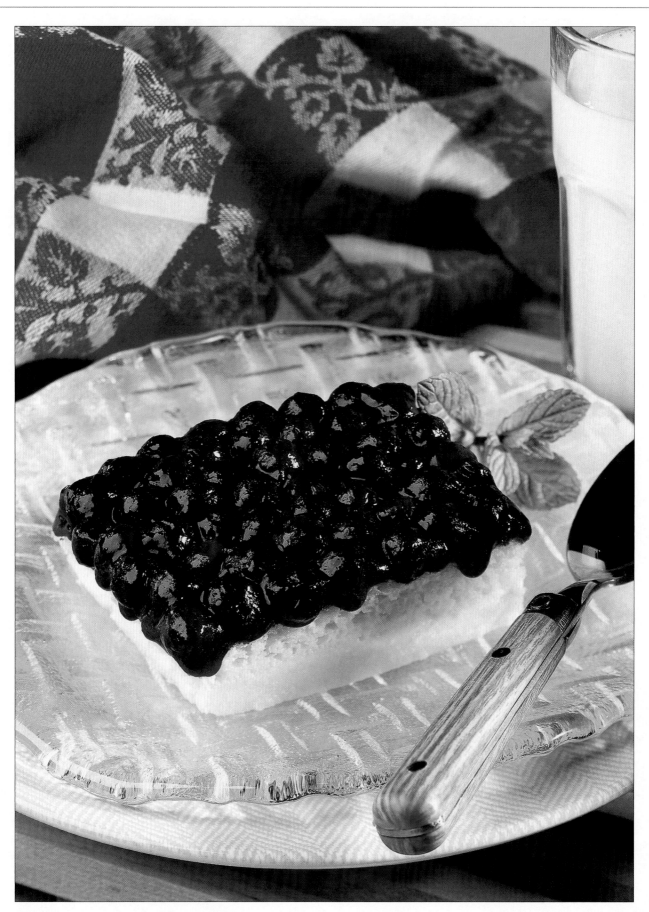

Blueberry Lemon Pudding Cake

Banana Chocolate Cupcakes

Makes 20 cupcakes

    2 cups all-purpose flour
    ¾ cup sugar, divided
    ¼ cup unsweetened cocoa powder
    ¾ teaspoon baking soda
    ½ teaspoon baking powder
    ¼ teaspoon salt
    8 ounces plain or banana low-fat yogurt
    ½ cup mashed ripe banana (1 medium banana)
    ⅓ cup canola or vegetable oil
    ¼ cup fat-free (skim) milk
    2 teaspoons vanilla extract
    3 egg whites
       Powdered Sugar Glaze (recipe follows)

Preheat oven to 350°F. Line 20 (2½-inch) muffin cups with foil baking cups.

Combine flour, ¼ cup sugar, cocoa, baking soda, baking powder and salt in large bowl; set aside. Blend yogurt, banana, oil, milk and vanilla in small bowl; mix well.

Beat egg whites at medium speed with electric mixer until foamy. Gradually add remaining ½ cup sugar, beating well after each addition, until sugar is dissolved and stiff peaks form. Stir yogurt mixture into flour mixture just until dry ingredients are moistened. Gently fold in ⅓ of egg white mixture until blended; fold in remaining egg white mixture. Fill muffin cups ⅔ full with batter.

Bake 20 to 25 minutes or until wooden pick inserted in centers comes out clean. Transfer cupcakes from pans to wire racks; cool completely. Drizzle Powdered Sugar Glaze over cupcakes; let stand until set. Store in airtight container at room temperature.

Powdered Sugar Glaze: Blend ½ cup powdered sugar and 1 tablespoon water in small bowl until smooth; add additional water, if necessary, to reach desired consistency.

Nutrients per serving: 1 cupcake
Calories: 138, Calories from Fat: 26%, Total Fat: 4g, Saturated Fat: <1g, Cholesterol: 1mg, Sodium: 109mg, Carbohydrate: 23g, Fiber: <1g, Protein: 3g

Dietary Exchanges: 1½ Starch, ½ Fat

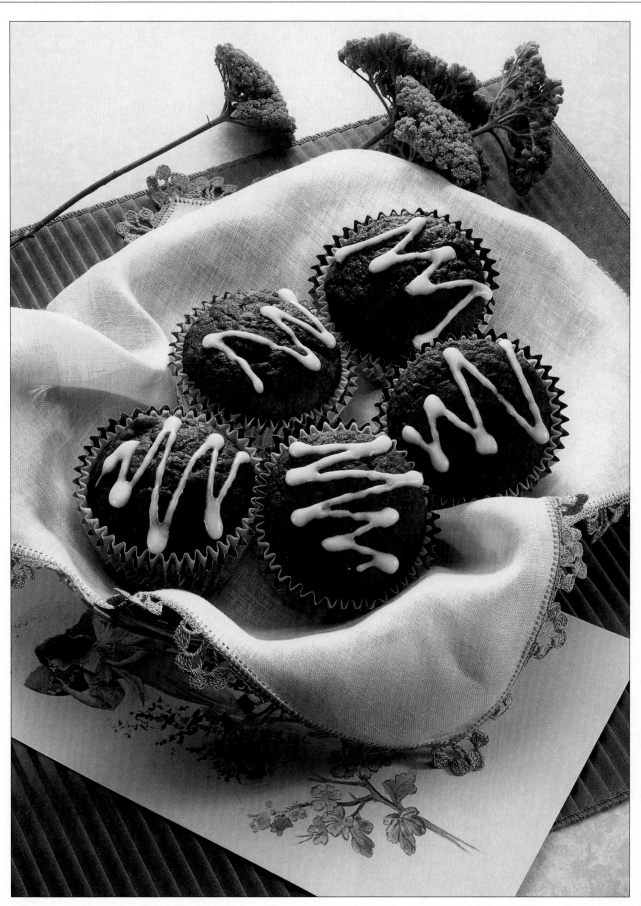

Banana Chocolate Cupcakes

Mixed Berry Cheesecake

Makes 16 servings

CRUST:
- 1½ cups fruit-juice-sweetened breakfast cereal flakes*
- 15 sugar-free low-fat butter-flavored cookies*
- 1 tablespoon vegetable oil

CHEESECAKE:
- 2 packages (8 ounces each) fat-free cream cheese, softened
- 2 cartons (8 ounces each) nonfat raspberry yogurt
- 1 package (8 ounces) Neufchâtel cream cheese, softened
- ½ cup all-fruit seedless blackberry preserves
- ½ cup all-fruit blueberry preserves
- 6 packages sugar substitute *or* equivalent of ¼ cup sugar
- 1 tablespoon vanilla
- ¼ cup water
- 1 package (0.3 ounces) sugar-free strawberry-flavored gelatin

TOPPING:
- 3 cups fresh or frozen unsweetened mixed berries, thawed

Available in the health food section of supermarkets.

Preheat oven to 400°F. Spray 10-inch springform pan with nonstick cooking spray.

To prepare crust, combine cereal, cookies and oil in food processor; process with on/off pulses until finely crushed. Press firmly onto bottom and ½ inch up side of pan. Bake 5 to 8 minutes or until crust is golden brown.

To prepare cheesecake, combine cream cheese, yogurt, Neufchâtel cheese, preserves, sugar substitute and vanilla in large bowl. Beat with electric mixer at high speed until smooth.

Combine water and gelatin in small microwavable bowl; microwave at HIGH 30 seconds to 1 minute or until water is boiling and gelatin is dissolved. Cool slightly. Add to cheese mixture; beat an additional 2 to 3 minutes or until well blended. Pour into springform pan; cover and refrigerate at least 24 hours. Top cheesecake with berries before serving.

Nutrients per serving: ¹⁄₁₆ of cheesecake
Calories: 186, Calories from Fat: 24%, Total Fat: 5g, Saturated Fat: 2g, Cholesterol: 11mg, Sodium: 290mg, Carbohydrate: 26g, Fiber: 2g, Protein: 8g

Dietary Exchanges: ½ Starch, 1½ Fruit, ¾ Meat, ½ Fat

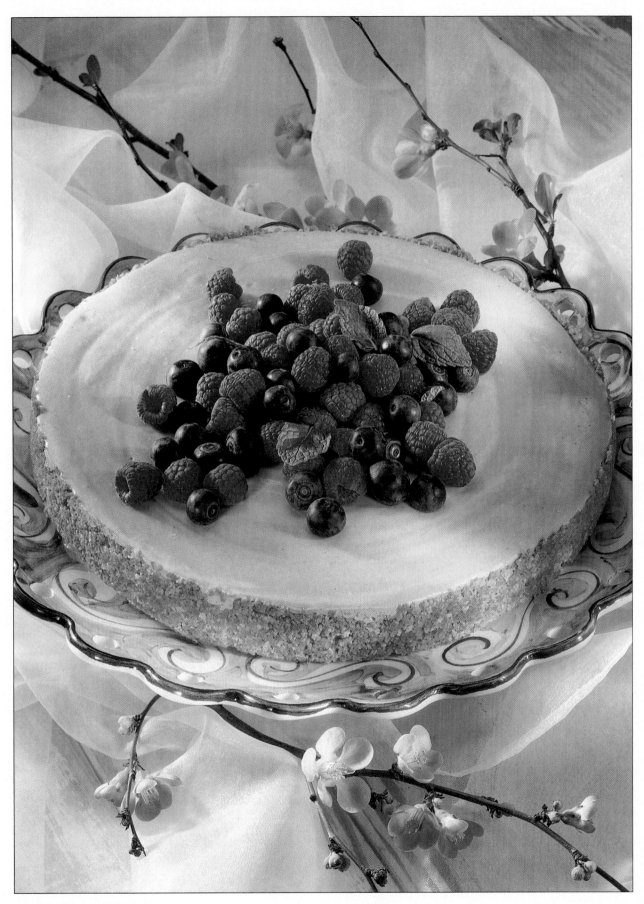

Mixed Berry Cheesecake

Raspberry Swirl Cheesecake

Makes 14 servings

> 2 tablespoons vanilla wafer cookie crumbs
> 2 containers (12 ounces each) nonfat cream cheese, softened
> ⅔ cup sugar
> 2 eggs
> 2 tablespoons cornstarch
> 2 teaspoons vanilla
> 1 cup low-fat sour cream
> 1 pint (2 cups) fresh raspberries, divided
> Mint sprigs for garnish

Preheat oven to 400°F. Coat bottom and 1 inch up side of 9-inch springform pan with nonstick cooking spray; coat with cookie crumbs. Beat cream cheese in large bowl with electric mixer until fluffy. Beat in sugar. Add eggs, cornstarch and vanilla; beat until smooth. Stir in sour cream until well combined. Pour batter into prepared pan.

Place 1 cup raspberries in food processor or blender; process until smooth. Strain purée; discard seeds. Spoon purée onto cheesecake; swirl into batter with knife.

Bake 45 to 50 minutes or until cheesecake is set around edge but slightly soft in center. Turn off oven; let cheesecake cool in oven about 3 hours, with oven door slightly opened.

Refrigerate cheesecake overnight. Remove side of pan; place cheesecake on serving plate. Garnish with remaining 1 cup raspberries and mint sprigs.

Nutrients per serving: 1/14 of cheesecake
Calories: 136, Calories from Fat: 19%, Total Fat: 3g, Saturated Fat: <1g, Cholesterol: 46mg, Sodium: 326mg, Carbohydrate: 17g, Fiber: <1g, Protein: 9g

Dietary Exchanges: 1 Starch, 1 Meat

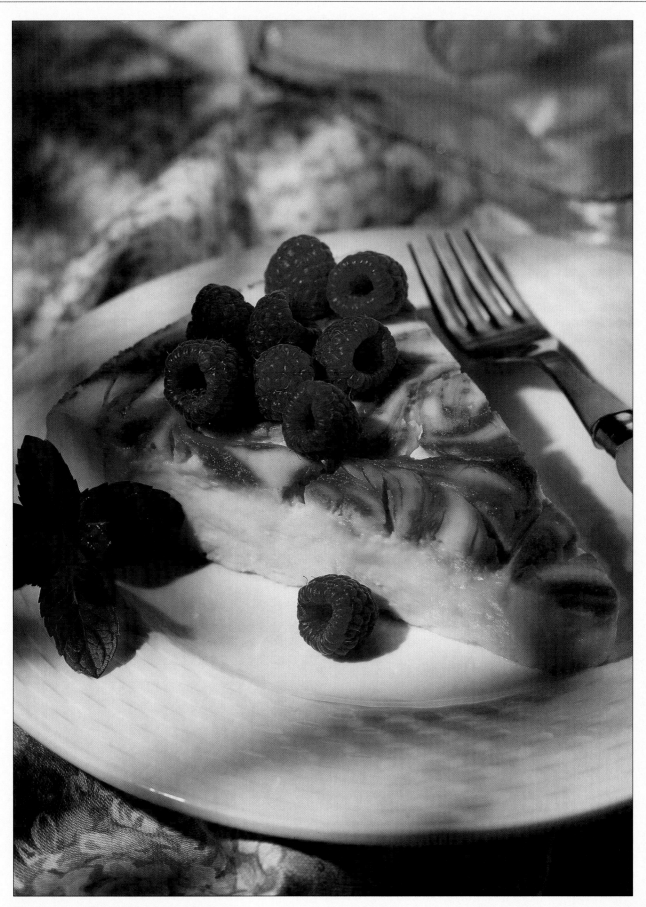

Raspberry Swirl Cheesecake

Low Fat Lemon Soufflé Cheesecake

Makes 8 servings

Prep Time: 15 minutes plus refrigerating

>   **1 graham cracker, crushed, divided**
> **⅔ cup boiling water**
>   **1 package (4-serving size) JELL-O® Brand Lemon Flavor
>   Sugar Free Low Calorie Gelatin Dessert**
>   **1 cup BREAKSTONE'S® *or* KNUDSEN® 2% Cottage Cheese**
>   **1 container (8 ounces) PHILADELPHIA FREE® Fat Free
>   Cream Cheese**
>   **2 cups thawed COOL WHIP FREE® Whipped Topping**

SPRINKLE ½ of the crumbs onto side of 8- or 9-inch springform pan or 9-inch pie plate which has been sprayed with no stick cooking spray.

STIR boiling water into gelatin in large bowl at least 2 minutes until completely dissolved. Pour into blender container. Add cheeses; cover. Blend on medium speed until smooth, scraping down sides occasionally.

POUR into large bowl. Gently stir in whipped topping. Pour into prepared pan; smooth top. Sprinkle remaining crumbs around outside edge.

REFRIGERATE 4 hours or until set. Remove side of pan just before serving. Garnish as desired. Store leftover cheesecake in refrigerator.

Nutrients per serving: ⅛ of cheesecake
Calories: 100, Calories from Fat: 18%, Total Fat: 2g, Saturated Fat: 1.5g, Cholesterol: 10mg, Sodium: 300mg, Carbohydrate: 11g, Fiber: 0g, Protein: 9g

Dietary Exchanges: 1 Starch, ½ Meat

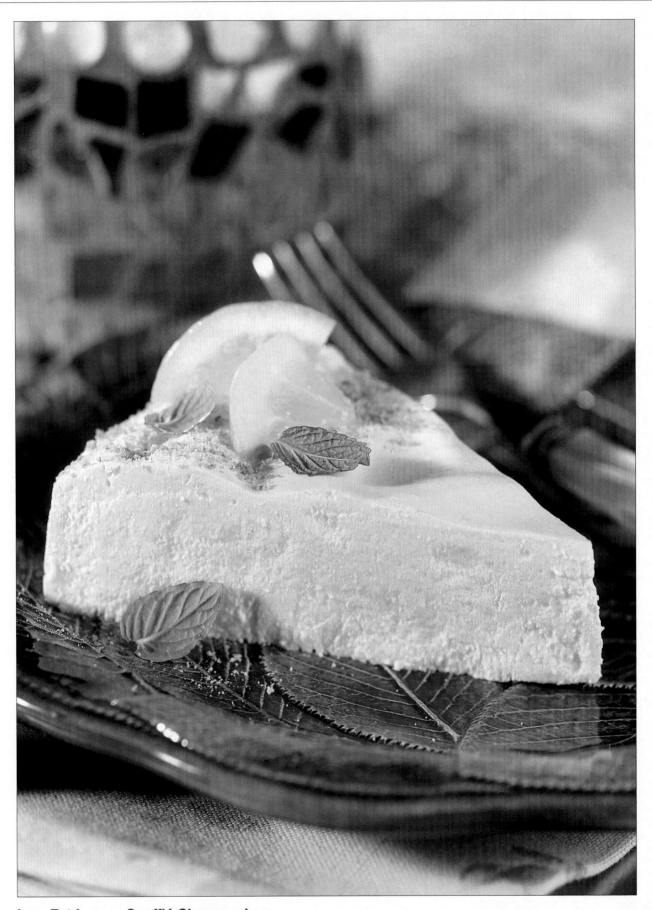

Low Fat Lemon Soufflé Cheesecake

Apricot Walnut Swirl Coffeecake

Makes 12 servings

> 2⅓ cups reduced-fat baking mix (BISQUICK®)
> 3½ teaspoons EQUAL® FOR RECIPES *or* 12 packets EQUAL®
>   sweetener *or* ½ cup EQUAL® SPOONFUL™
> ⅔ cup skim milk
> ⅓ cup fat-free sour cream
> 1 egg
> 2 tablespoons melted margarine
>   Apricot Walnut Filling (recipe follows)
> ⅓ cup light apricot preserves sweetened with NutraSweet®
>   brand sweetener or apricot spreadable fruit

Combine baking mix and Equal®; mix in milk, sour cream, egg and margarine. Spread ⅓ of batter in greased and floured 6-cup Bundt pan; spoon half the filling over batter. Repeat layers, ending with batter.

Bake in preheated 375°F oven until coffeecake is browned on top and toothpick inserted in center comes out clean, about 25 minutes. Cool in pan 5 minutes; invert onto rack and cool 5 to 10 minutes.

Spoon apricot preserves over top of coffeecake; serve warm.

Apricot Walnut Filling

> ½ cup light apricot preserves sweetened with NutraSweet®
>   brand sweetener or apricot spreadable fruit
> 5½ teaspoons EQUAL® FOR RECIPES *or* 18 packets EQUAL®
>   sweetener *or* ¾ cup EQUAL® SPOONFUL™
> 4 teaspoons ground cinnamon
> ½ cup chopped walnuts

Mix all ingredients in small bowl.

Nutrients per serving: 1/12 of cheesecake
Calories: 189, Calories from Fat: 34%, Total Fat: 7g, Saturated Fat: 1g, Cholesterol: 18mg, Sodium: 332mg, Carbohydrate: 28g, Fiber: 1g, Protein: 4g

Dietary Exchanges: 2 Starch, 1 Fat

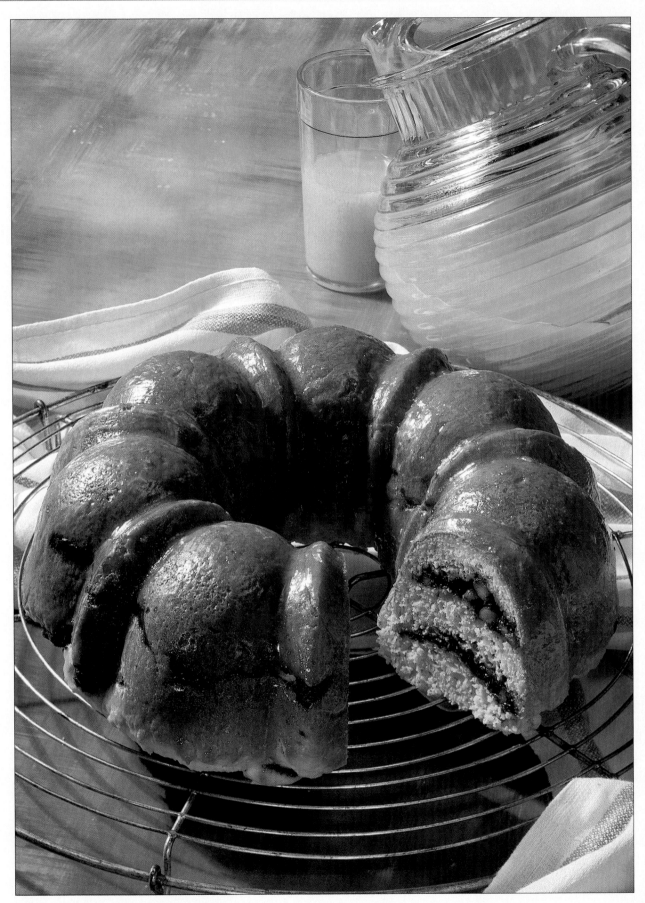

Apricot Walnut Swirl Coffeecake

Pineapple Upside-Down Cake

Makes 8 servings

1 can (14 ounces) unsweetened crushed pineapple in juice, undrained
¼ cup pecan pieces (optional)
2 tablespoons lemon juice
1¾ teaspoons EQUAL® FOR RECIPES *or* 6 packets EQUAL® sweetener *or* ¼ cup EQUAL® SPOONFUL™
1 teaspoon cornstarch
4 tablespoons margarine, at room temperature
3½ teaspoons EQUAL® FOR RECIPES *or* 12 packets EQUAL® sweetener *or* ½ cup EQUAL® SPOONFUL™
1 egg
1 cup cake flour
1½ teaspoons baking powder
½ teaspoon baking soda
¼ teaspoon ground cinnamon
¼ teaspoon ground nutmeg
⅛ teaspoon ground ginger
⅓ cup buttermilk

Drain pineapple, reserving ¼ cup juice. Mix pineapple, pecans, 1 tablespoon lemon juice, 1¾ teaspoons Equal® For Recipes or 6 packets Equal® sweetener or ¼ cup Equal® Spoonful™ and cornstarch in bottom of 8-inch square or 9-inch round cake pan; spread mixture evenly in pan.

Beat margarine and 3½ teaspoons Equal® For Recipes or 12 packets Equal® sweetener or ½ cup Equal® Spoonful™ in medium bowl until fluffy; beat in egg. Combine flour, baking powder, baking soda and spices in small bowl. Add to margarine mixture alternately with buttermilk, ¼ cup reserved pineapple juice and remaining 1 tablespoon lemon juice, beginning and ending with dry ingredients. Spread batter over pineapple mixture in cake pan.

Bake in preheated 350°F oven until browned and toothpick inserted in center comes out clean, about 25 minutes. Invert cake immediately onto serving plate. Serve warm or at room temperature. If desired, maraschino cherry halves may be placed in bottom of cake pan with pineapple mixture.

Nutrients per serving: ⅛ of cake
Calories: 155, Calories from Fat: 38%, Total Fat: 7g, Saturated Fat: 1g, Cholesterol: 27mg, Sodium: 256mg, Carbohydrate: 22g, Fiber: 1g, Protein: 3g

Dietary Exchanges: 1 Starch, ½ Fruit, ½ Fat

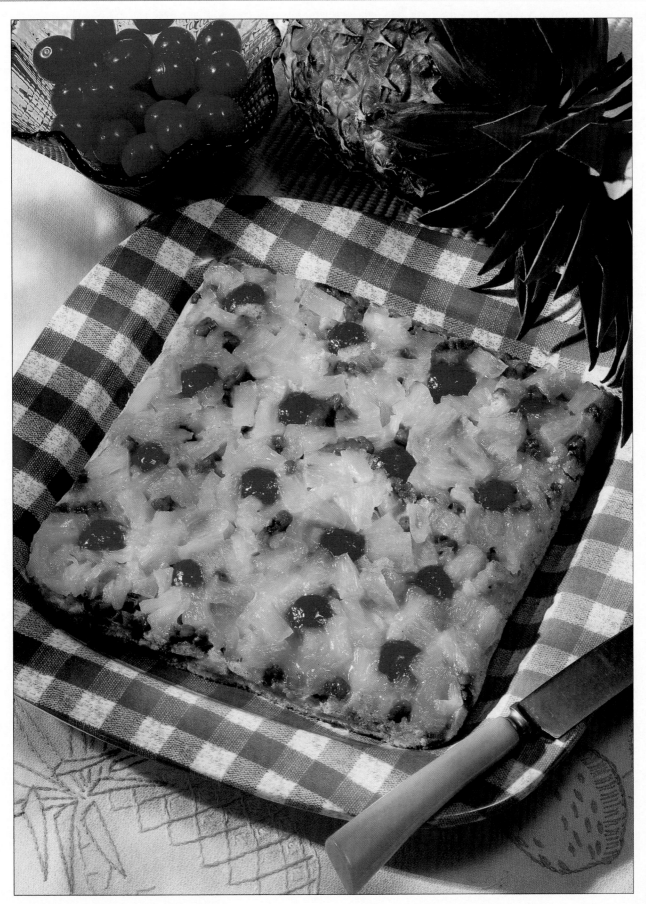

Pineapple Upside-Down Cake

Luscious Chocolate Cheesecake

Makes 12 servings

> 2 cups (1 pound) nonfat cottage cheese
> ¾ cup liquid egg substitute
> ⅔ cup sugar
> 4 ounces (½ of 8-ounce package) Neufchâtel cheese (⅓ less fat cream cheese), softened
> ⅓ cup HERSHEY¡S Cocoa or HERSHEY¡S Dutch Processed Cocoa
> ½ teaspoon vanilla extract
> Yogurt Topping (recipe follows)
> Sliced strawberries or mandarin orange segments (optional)

Heat oven to 300°F. Spray 9-inch springform pan with vegetable cooking spray.

Place cottage cheese, egg substitute, sugar, Neufchâtel cheese, cocoa and vanilla in food processor; process until smooth. Pour into prepared pan. Bake 35 minutes or until edges are set.

Meanwhile, prepare Yogurt Topping. Carefully spread topping over cheesecake. Continue baking 5 minutes. Remove from oven to wire rack. With knife, loosen cheesecake from side of pan. Cool completely.

Cover; refrigerate until chilled. Remove side of pan. Serve with strawberries or mandarin orange segments, if desired. Refrigerate leftover cheesecake.

Yogurt Topping

> ⅔ cup plain nonfat yogurt
> 2 tablespoons sugar

Stir together yogurt and sugar in small bowl until well blended.

Nutrients per serving: $1/12$ of cheesecake
Calories: 84, Calories from Fat: 27%, Total Fat: 2g, Saturated Fat: 1g, Cholesterol: 7mg, Sodium: 199mg, Carbohydrate: 6g, Fiber: 1g, Protein: 8g

Dietary Exchanges: ½ Starch; 1 Meat

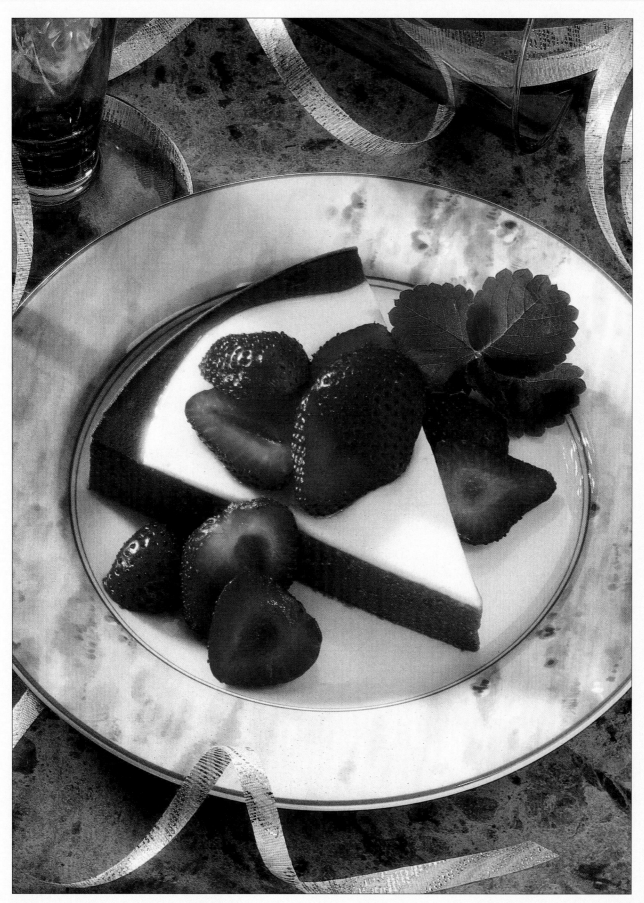

Luscious Chocolate Cheesecake

pies & tarts

Country Peach Tart

Makes 8 servings

> **Pastry for single crust 9-inch pie**
> **1 tablespoon all-purpose flour**
> **2½ teaspoons EQUAL® FOR RECIPES** *or* **8 packets EQUAL®**
> **sweetener** *or* **⅓ cup EQUAL® SPOONFUL™**
> **4 cups sliced pitted peeled fresh peaches (about 4 medium)**
> **or frozen peaches, thawed**
> **Ground nutmeg**

Roll pastry on floured surface into 12-inch circle; transfer to ungreased cookie sheet. Combine flour and Equal®; sprinkle over peaches and toss. Arrange peaches on pastry, leaving 2-inch border around edge of pastry. Sprinkle peaches lightly with nutmeg. Bring pastry edge toward center, overlapping as necessary.

Bake tart in preheated 425°F oven until crust is browned and fruit is tender, 25 to 30 minutes.

Nutrients per serving: ⅛ of tart
Calories: 201, Calories from Fat: 31%, Total Fat: 7g, Saturated Fat: 3g, Cholesterol: 5mg, Sodium: 100mg, Carbohydrate: 34g, Fiber: 3g, Protein: 2g

Dietary Exchanges: 1 Starch, 1 Fruit, 1½ Fat

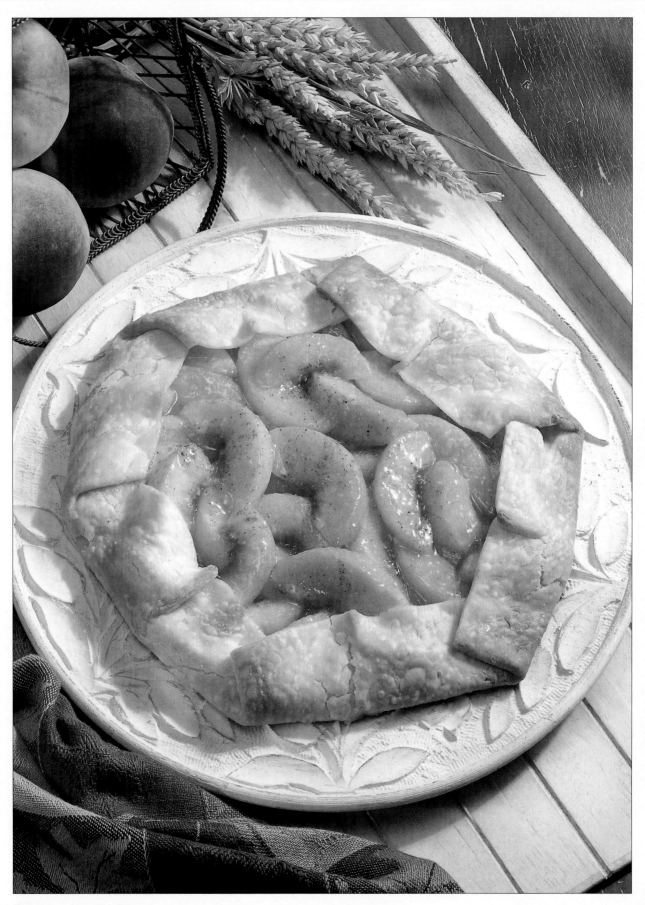

Country Peach Tart

Strawberry Cream Pie

Makes 8 servings

> 1 package (8 ounces) reduced-fat cream cheese, softened
> 1¾ teaspoons EQUAL® FOR RECIPES *or* 6 packets EQUAL® sweetener *or* ¼ cup EQUAL® SPOONFUL™
> 1 teaspoon vanilla
> Reduced-fat graham cracker crust (9 inch) or homemade graham cracker crust
> 1 cup cold water
> 2 tablespoons cornstarch
> 1 package (0.3 ounces) sugar-free strawberry gelatin
> 3½ teaspoons EQUAL® FOR RECIPES *or* 12 packets EQUAL® sweetener *or* ½ cup EQUAL® SPOONFUL™
> 1 pint strawberries, hulled and sliced
> 8 tablespoons frozen light whipped topping (optional)

Beat cream cheese, 1¾ teaspoons Equal® for Recipes and vanilla in small bowl until fluffy; spread evenly in bottom of crust. Mix cold water and cornstarch in small saucepan; heat to boiling, whisking constantly until thickened, about 1 minute. Add gelatin and 3½ teaspoons Equal® for Recipes, whisking until gelatin is dissolved. Cool 10 minutes.

Arrange half of strawberries over cream cheese; spoon half of gelatin mixture over strawberries. Arrange remaining strawberries over pie and spoon remaining gelatin mixture over strawberries.

Refrigerate until pie is set and chilled, 1 to 2 hours. Serve with whipped topping, if desired.

Nutrients per serving: ⅛ of pie
Calories: 185, Calories from Fat: 40%, Total Fat: 8g, Saturated Fat: 4g, Cholesterol: 13mg, Sodium: 246mg, Carbohydrate: 22g, Fiber: 1g, Protein: 4g

Dietary Exchanges: 1 Starch, ½ Fruit, 1½ Fat

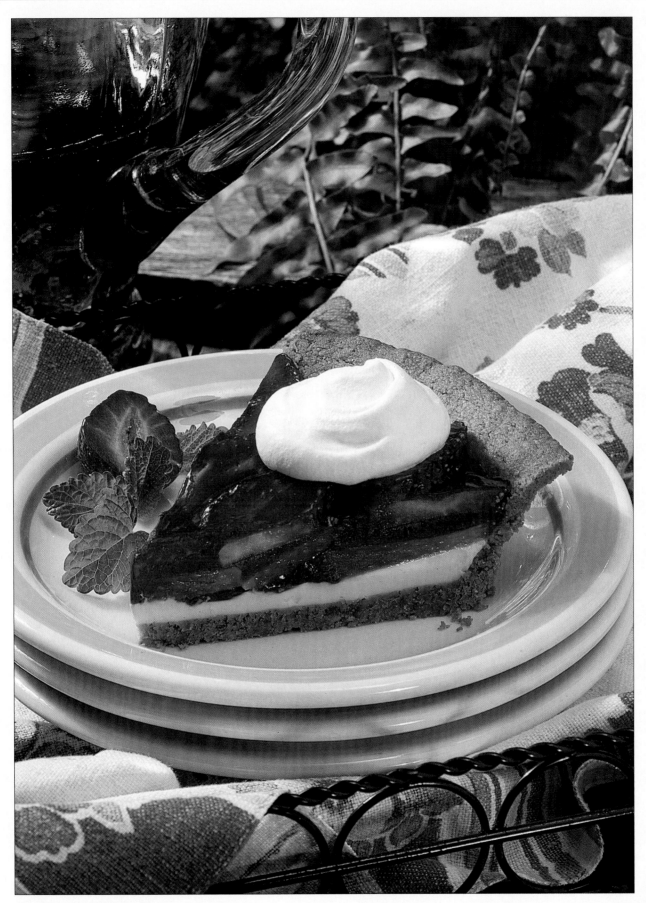

Strawberry Cream Pie

Key Lime Tarts

Makes 8 servings

¾ **cup fat-free (skim) milk**
6 **tablespoons fresh lime juice**
2 **tablespoons cornstarch**
½ **cup cholesterol-free egg substitute**
½ **cup reduced-fat sour cream**
12 **packages sugar substitute** *or* **equivalent of ½ cup sugar**
  Butter-flavored nonstick cooking spray
4 **sheets phyllo dough***
¾ **cup thawed frozen fat-free nondairy whipped topping**

*Cover with damp kitchen towel to prevent dough from drying out.

Combine milk, lime juice and cornstarch in medium saucepan. Cook over medium heat 2 to 3 minutes, stirring constantly until thick. Remove from heat.

Add egg substitute; whisk constantly for 30 seconds to allow egg substitute to cook. Stir in sour cream and sugar substitute; cover and refrigerate until cool.

Preheat oven to 350°F. Spray 8 (2½-inch) muffin cups with cooking spray; set aside.

Place 1 sheet of phyllo dough on cutting board; spray with cooking spray. Top with second sheet of phyllo dough; spray with cooking spray. Top with third sheet of phyllo dough; spray with cooking spray. Top with last sheet; spray with cooking spray.

Cut stack of phyllo dough into 8 squares. Gently fit each stacked square into prepared muffin cup; press firmly against bottom and side. Bake 8 to 10 minutes or until golden brown. Carefully remove from muffin cups; cool on wire rack.

Divide lime mixture evenly among phyllo cups; top with whipped topping. Garnish with fresh raspberries and lime slices, if desired.

Nutrients per serving: 1 tart
Calories: 82, Calories from Fat: 17%, Total Fat: 1g, Saturated Fat: <1g, Cholesterol: 5mg, Sodium: 88mg, Carbohydrate: 13g, Fiber: <1g, Protein: 3g

Dietary Exchanges: 1 Starch

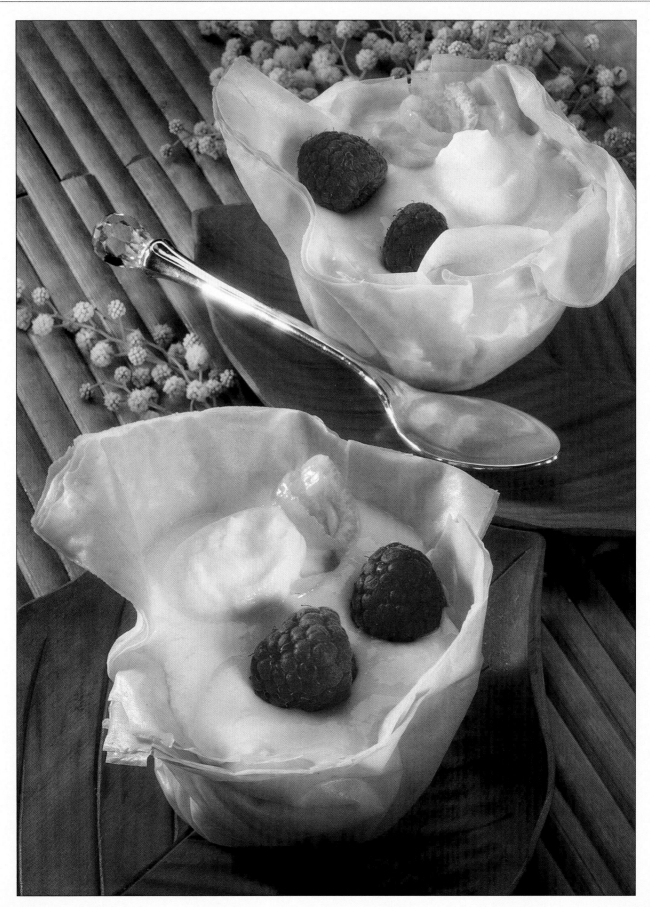

Key Lime Tarts

Oats 'n' Apple Tart

Makes 8 servings

- 1½ cups uncooked quick oats
- ½ cup brown sugar, divided
- 1 tablespoon plus ¼ teaspoon ground cinnamon, divided
- 5 tablespoons butter or margarine, melted
- 2 medium sweet apples, such as Golden Delicious, unpeeled, cored and thinly sliced
- 1 teaspoon lemon juice
- ¼ cup water
- 1 envelope unsweetened gelatin
- ½ cup apple juice concentrate
- 1 package (8 ounces) reduced-fat cream cheese, softened
- ⅛ teaspoon ground nutmeg

Preheat oven to 350°F. Combine oats, ¼ cup brown sugar and 1 tablespoon cinnamon in medium bowl; stir. Add butter and stir until combined. Press into bottom and up sides of 9-inch pie plate. Bake 7 minutes or until set. Cool on wire rack.

Toss apple slices with lemon juice in small bowl; set aside. Place water in small saucepan. Sprinkle gelatin over water; let stand 3 to 5 minutes. Stir in apple juice concentrate. Cook and stir over medium heat until gelatin is dissolved. *Do not boil.* Remove from heat and set aside.

Beat cream cheese on medium speed of electric mixer in medium bowl until fluffy and smooth. Add remaining ¼ cup brown sugar, ¼ teaspoon cinnamon and nutmeg. Mix until smooth. Slowly beat in gelatin mixture on low speed until blended and creamy, about 1 minute. *Do not overbeat.*

Arrange apple slices in crust. Pour cream cheese mixture evenly over top. Refrigerate 2 hours or until set. Garnish as desired.

Nutrients per serving: ⅛ of tart
Calories: 245, Calories from Fat: 48%, Total Fat: 13g, Saturated Fat: 8g, Cholesterol: 34mg, Sodium: 221mg, Carbohydrate: 26g, Fiber: 3g, Protein: 6g

Dietary Exchanges: 1 Starch, 1 Fruit, 2½ Fat

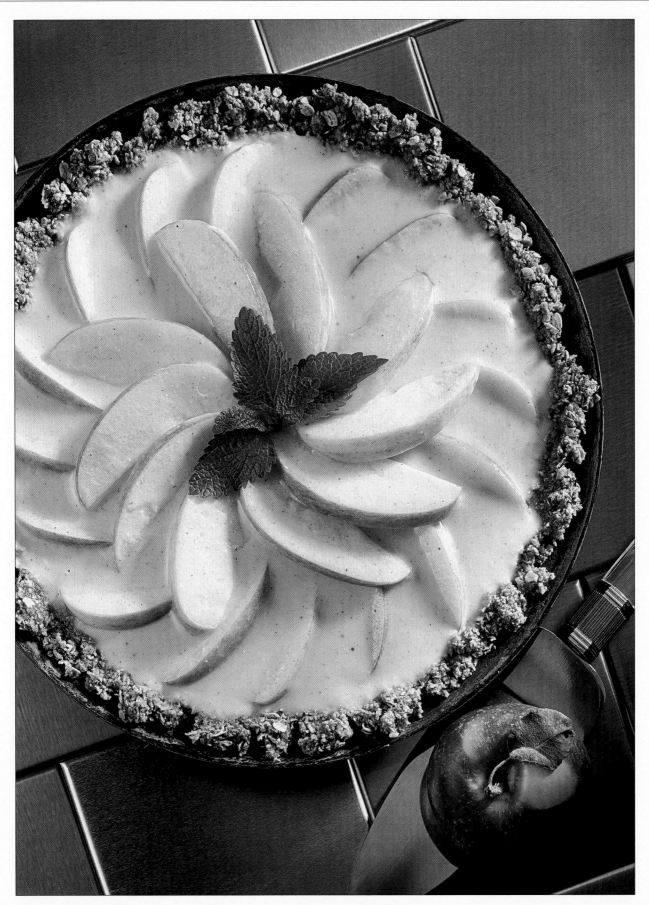

Oats 'n' Apple Tart

Pumpkin Pie

Makes 8 servings

> **Pastry for single crust 9-inch pie**
> 1 can (16 ounces) pumpkin
> 1 can (12 ounces) evaporated skim milk
> 3 eggs
> 5½ teaspoons **EQUAL® FOR RECIPES** *or* **18 packets EQUAL®**
> **sweetener** *or* ¾ cup **EQUAL® SPOONFUL™**
> 1 teaspoon ground cinnamon
> ½ teaspoon ground ginger
> ¼ teaspoon salt
> ¼ teaspoon ground nutmeg
> ⅛ teaspoon ground cloves

Roll pastry on floured surface into circle 1 inch larger than inverted 9-inch pie pan. Ease pastry into pan; trim and flute edge.

Beat pumpkin, evaporated milk and eggs in medium bowl; beat in remaining ingredients. Pour into pastry shell. Bake in preheated 425°F oven 15 minutes; reduce heat to 350°F and bake until knife inserted near center comes out clean, about 40 minutes. Cool on wire rack.

Nutrients per serving:
Calories: 214, Calories from Fat: 39%, Total Fat: 9g, Saturated Fat: 4g, Cholesterol: 87mg, Sodium: 254mg, Carbohydrate: 26g, Fiber: 2g, Protein: 7g

Dietary Exchanges: 2 Starch, 1½ Fat

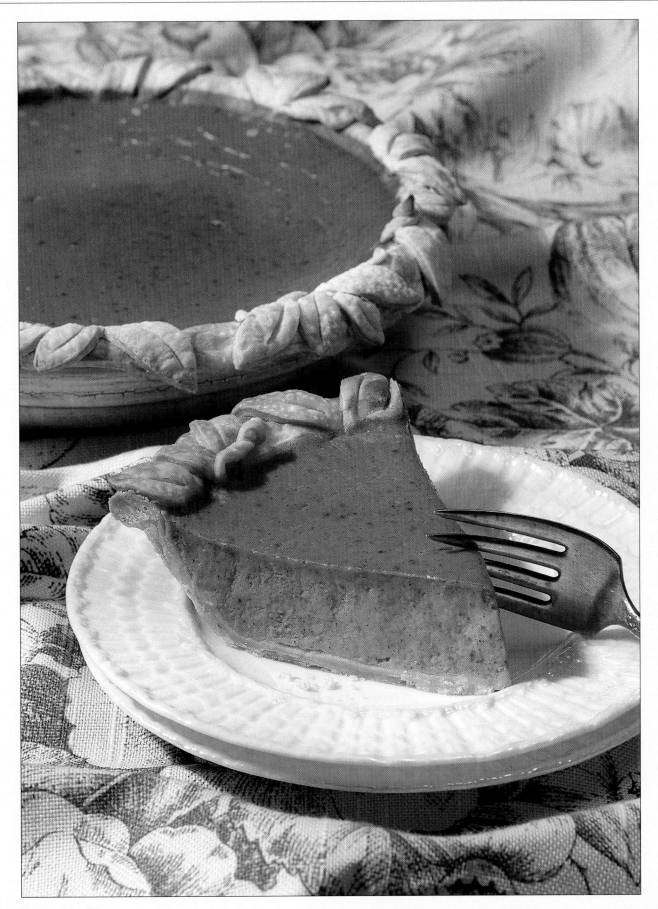

Pumpkin Pie

Apple-Cranberry Tart

Makes 12 servings

1⅓ cups all-purpose flour
¾ cup plus 1 tablespoon sugar, divided
¼ teaspoon salt
2 tablespoons vegetable shortening
2 tablespoons margarine
4 to 5 tablespoons ice water
⅓ cup dried cranberries
½ cup boiling water
1 teaspoon ground cinnamon
2 tablespoons cornstarch
4 medium baking apples
Vanilla frozen yogurt (optional)

Combine flour, 1 tablespoon sugar and salt in medium bowl. Cut in shortening and margarine with pastry blender or two knives until mixture forms coarse crumbs. Mix in ice water, 1 tablespoon at a time, until mixture comes together and forms soft dough. Wrap in plastic wrap. Refrigerate 30 minutes.

Combine cranberries and boiling water in small bowl. Let stand 20 minutes or until softened. Preheat oven to 425°F. Roll out dough on floured surface to ⅛-inch thickness. Cut into 11-inch circle. (Reserve any leftover dough scraps for decorating top of tart.) Ease dough into 10-inch tart pan with removable bottom, leaving ¼-inch dough above rim of pan. Prick bottom and sides of dough with tines of fork; bake 12 minutes or until dough begins to brown. Cool on wire rack. *Reduce oven temperature to 375°F.*

Combine remaining ¾ cup sugar and cinnamon in large bowl; mix well. Reserve 1 teaspoon mixture. Add cornstarch to bowl; mix well. Peel, core and thinly slice apples, adding pieces to bowl as they are sliced; toss well. Drain cranberries; add to apple mixture and toss well.

Arrange apple mixture attractively over dough. Sprinkle reserved 1 teaspoon sugar mixture evenly over top of tart. Place tart on baking sheet; bake 30 to 35 minutes or until apples are tender and crust is golden brown. Cool on wire rack. Remove side of pan; place tart on serving plate. Serve warm or at room temperature.

Nutrients per serving: ¹⁄₁₂ of tart
Calories: 175, Calories from Fat: 21%, Total Fat: 4g, Saturated Fat: 1g, Cholesterol: <1mg, Sodium: 45mg, Carbohydrate: 33g, Fiber: 1g, Protein: 1g

Dietary Exchanges: 1 Starch, 1 Fruit, 1 Fat

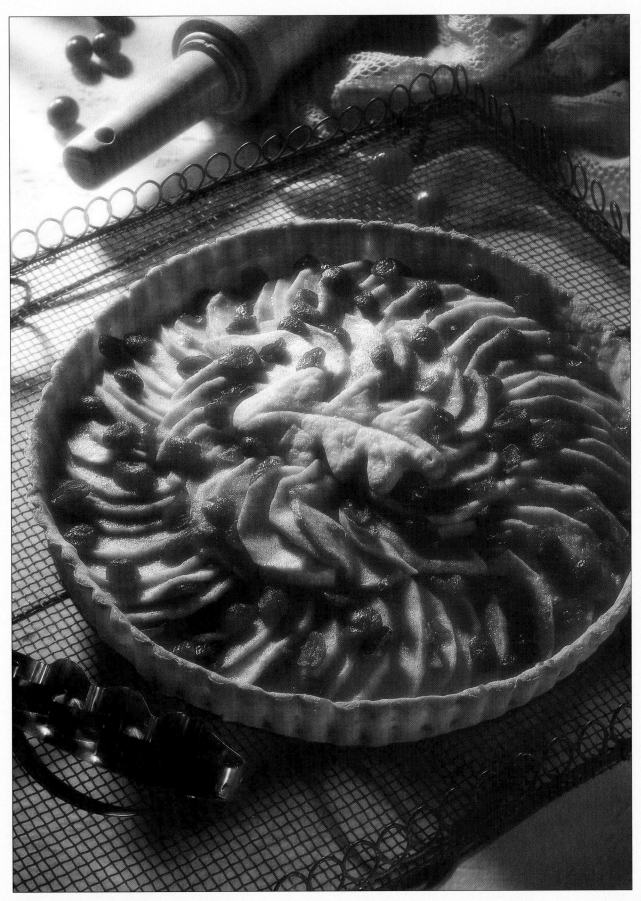

Apple-Cranberry Tart

classic
favorites

Berries with Banana Cream

Makes 2 servings

⅓ cup reduced-fat sour cream
½ small ripe banana, cut into chunks
1 tablespoon frozen orange juice concentrate
**2 cups sliced strawberries, blueberries, raspberries or
  a combination**
Ground cinnamon or nutmeg

Combine sour cream, banana and juice concentrate in blender. Cover and blend until smooth.

Place berries in two serving dishes. Top with sour cream mixture. Sprinkle with cinnamon.

Nutrients per serving: 1 berry cup + ½ of sour cream mixture
Calories: 135, Calories from Fat: 25%, Total Fat: 4g, Saturated Fat: 3g, Cholesterol: 13mg, Sodium: 29mg, Carbohydrate: 23g, Fiber: 4g, Protein: 4g

Dietary Exchanges: 1½ Fruit, 1 Fat

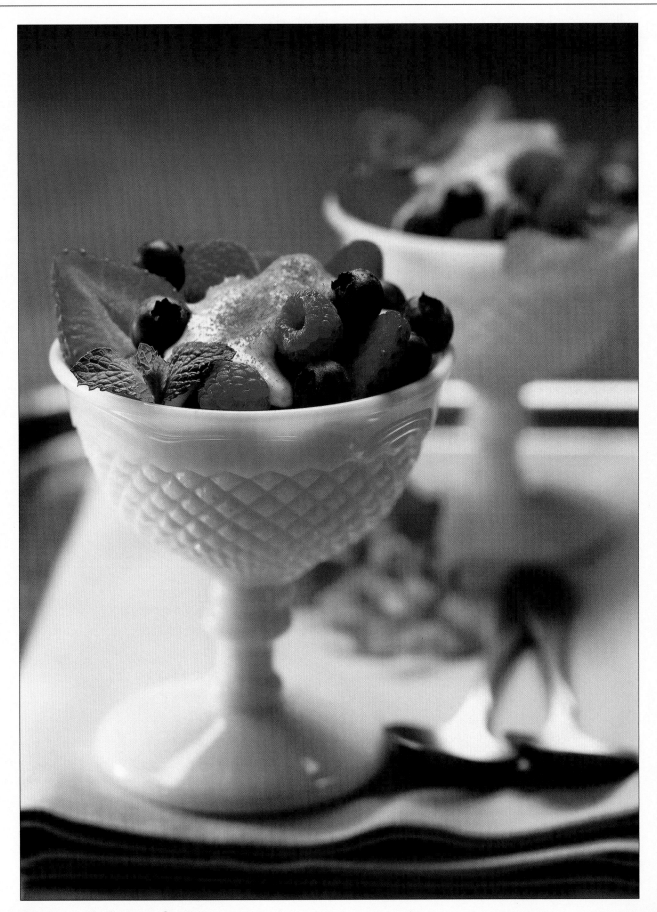

Berries with Banana Cream

Peach Melba Dessert

Makes 15 servings

Prep Time: 15 minutes plus refrigerating

        1½ **cups boiling water**
          1 **package (8-serving size)** *or* **2 packages (4-serving size**
                 each) JELL-O® Brand Raspberry Flavor Sugar Free Low
                 Calorie Gelatin
          2 **cups cold apple juice**
        1½ **cups graham cracker crumbs**
          ½ **cup sugar, divided**
          ½ **cup (1 stick) margarine, melted**
          1 **package (8 ounces) PHILADELPHIA® Neufchâtel Cheese,**
                 ⅓ **Less Fat than Cream Cheese, softened**
          1 **tub (8 ounces) COOL WHIP FREE® Whipped Topping,**
                 thawed
          1 **can (16 ounces) sliced peaches, drained**
          1 **cup raspberries**

STIR boiling water into gelatin in large bowl at least 2 minutes until completely dissolved. Stir in apple juice. Refrigerate about 1½ hours or until thickened (spoon drawn through leaves definite impression).

MEANWHILE, mix crumbs, ¼ cup of the sugar and margarine in 13×9-inch pan. Press firmly onto bottom of pan. Refrigerate until ready to fill.

BEAT cheese and remaining ¼ cup sugar in large bowl until smooth. Gently stir in 2 cups of the whipped topping. Spread evenly over crust. Arrange peaches and raspberries on cheese mixture. Spoon gelatin over cheese layer.

REFRIGERATE 3 hours or until firm. Serve with remaining whipped topping.

Nutrients per serving: 1/15 of dessert
Calories: 210, Calories from Fat: 47%, Total Fat: 11g, Saturated Fat: 5g, Cholesterol: 10mg, Sodium: 220mg, Carbohydrate: 26g, Fiber: 1g, Protein: 3g

Dietary Exchanges: 2 Starch, 2 Fat

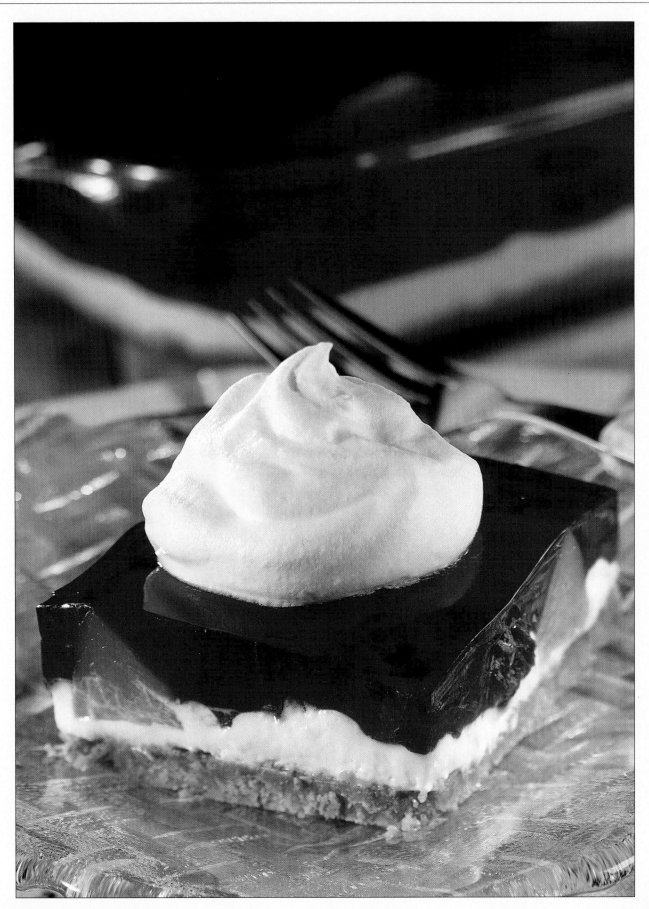

Peach Melba Dessert

classicfavorites

Chocolate-Strawberry Crêpes

Makes 8 servings (2 crêpes each)

CRÊPES
- ⅔ cup all-purpose flour
- 2 tablespoons unsweetened cocoa powder
- 6 packages sugar substitute *or* equivalent of ¼ cup sugar
- ¼ teaspoon salt
- 1¼ cups fat-free (skim) milk
- ½ cup cholesterol-free egg substitute
- 1 tablespoon margarine, melted
- 1 teaspoon vanilla
- Nonstick cooking spray

FILLING AND TOPPING
- 4 ounces fat-free cream cheese, softened
- 1 package (1.3 ounces) chocolate-fudge-flavored sugar-free instant pudding mix
- 1½ cups fat-free (skim) milk
- ¼ cup all-fruit strawberry preserves
- 2 tablespoons water
- 2 cups fresh hulled and quartered strawberries

For crêpes, combine flour, cocoa, sugar substitute and salt in food processor; process to blend. Add milk, egg substitute, margarine and vanilla; process until smooth. Let stand at room temperature 30 minutes.

Spray 7-inch nonstick skillet with cooking spray; heat over medium-high heat. Pour 2 tablespoons batter into hot pan. Immediately rotate pan back and forth to swirl batter over entire surface of pan. Cook 1 to 2 minutes or until brown around edge and top is dry. Carefully turn with spatula; cook 30 seconds more. Transfer to waxed paper. Repeat with remaining batter. Separate crêpes with sheets of waxed paper.

For chocolate filling, beat cream cheese in medium bowl with electric mixer at high speed until smooth; set aside. Prepare chocolate pudding with skim milk. Gradually add to cream cheese mixture; beat at high 3 minutes. For strawberry topping, combine preserves and water in large bowl until smooth. Add strawberries; toss to coat. Spread 2 tablespoons chocolate filling evenly over surface of crêpe; roll tightly. Top with strawberries. Garnish as desired. Serve immediately.

Nutrients per serving: 2 crêpes
Calories: 161, Calories from Fat: 13%, Total Fat: 2g, Saturated Fat: <1g, Cholesterol: 1mg, Sodium: 374mg, Carbohydrate: 27g, Fiber: 1g, Protein: 8g

Dietary Exchanges: 2 Fruit

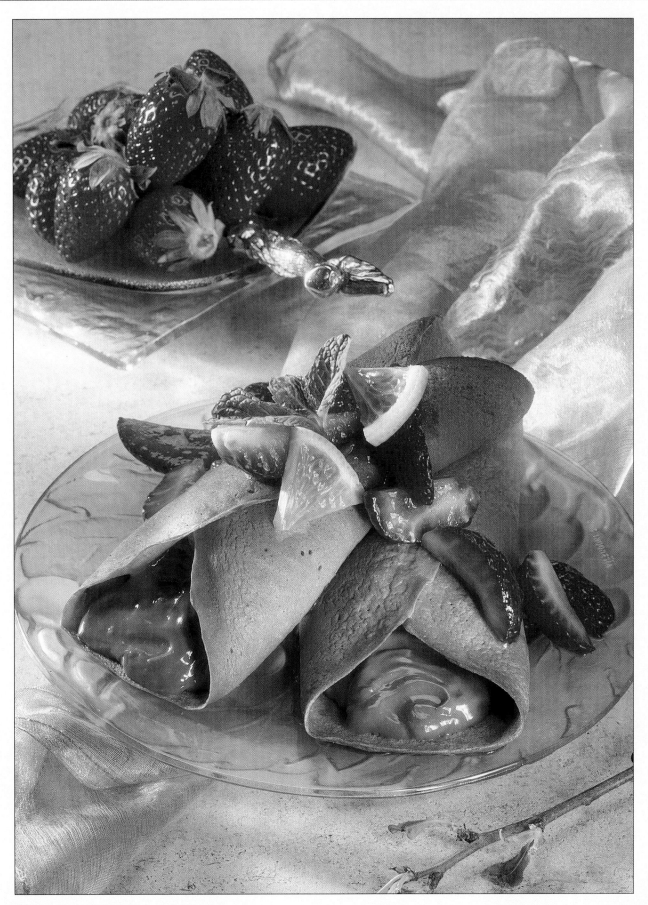

Chocolate-Strawberry Crêpes

Better Banana Bread

Makes 1 loaf (8½×4 inches, 14 slices) or 3 loaves (5⅝×3¼ inches)

> 1 cup mashed very ripe bananas (about 3 small)
> ½ cup plain fat-free yogurt
> 4 tablespoons margarine, melted
> 1 egg
> 1 egg white
> 7¼ teaspoons EQUAL® FOR RECIPES *or* 24 packets EQUAL®
>   sweetener *or* 1 cup EQUAL® SPOONFUL™
> 1 teaspoon vanilla
> 2 cups all-purpose flour
> 1 teaspoon baking powder
> ½ teaspoon baking soda
> ¼ teaspoon salt
> ¼ to ½ cup walnut pieces (optional)

Beat banana, yogurt, margarine, egg, egg white, Equal® and vanilla at medium speed in large bowl until blended; beat at high speed 1 minute. Add combined flour, baking powder, baking soda and salt, mixing just until ingredients are moistened. Stir in walnuts, if desired.

Pour batter into one 8½×4-inch greased and floured loaf pan or three 5⅝×3¼-inch loaf pans. Bake in preheated 350°F oven until bread is golden and toothpick inserted in center comes out clean, 55 to 65 minutes for large loaf, 35 to 40 minutes for small loaves. Cool 10 minutes in pan on wire rack; remove from pan and cool completely.

Nutrients per serving: ¼ slice of 8½×4-inch loaf
Calories: 123, Calories from Fat: 28%, Total Fat: 4g, Saturated Fat: 1g, Cholesterol: 15mg, Sodium: 175mg, Carbohydrate: 19g, Fiber: 1g, Protein: 3g

Dietary Exchanges: 1 Starch, 1 Fat

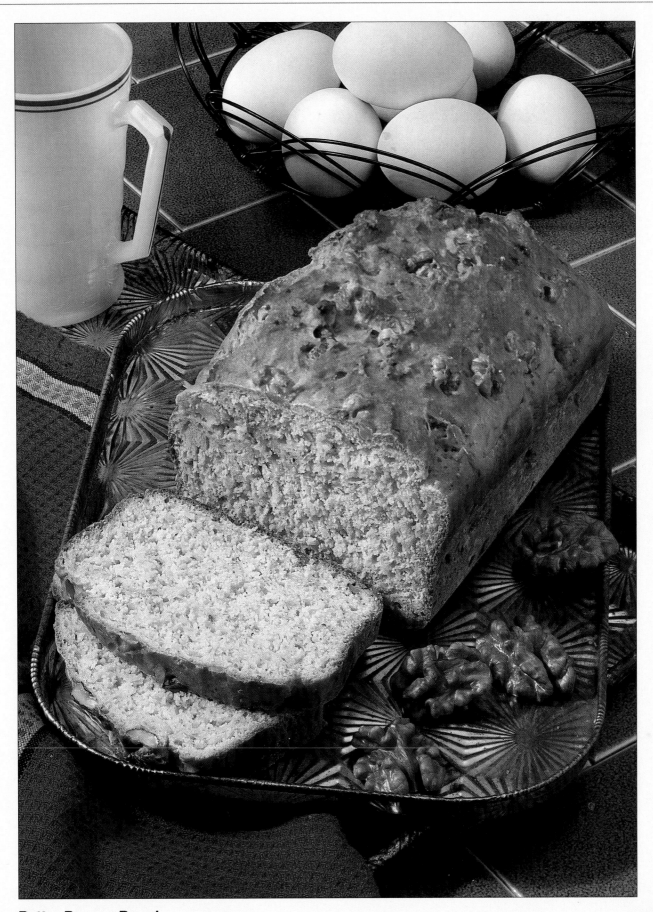

Better Banana Bread

Bittersweet Chocolate Torte

Makes 12 servings

> **6 tablespoons margarine**
> **⅓ cup skim milk**
> **⅓ cup apricot preserves with NutraSweet® brand sweetener or apricot spreadable fruit**
> **4 ounces unsweetened chocolate**
> **2 teaspoons instant espresso coffee crystals**
> **1 egg yolk**
> **1 teaspoon vanilla**
> **10¾ teaspoons EQUAL® FOR RECIPES *or* 36 packets EQUAL® sweetener *or* 1½ cups EQUAL® SPOONFUL™**
> **3 egg whites**
> **⅛ teaspoon cream of tartar**
> **¼ cup all-purpose flour**
> **⅛ teaspoon salt**
> **Rich Chocolate Glaze (optional, recipe follows)**
> **Light whipped topping, chocolate drizzle and/or raspberries (optional)**

Lightly grease bottom of 9-inch round cake pan and line with parchment or baking paper. Heat margarine, milk, apricot preserves, chocolate and espresso crystals in small saucepan, whisking frequently, until chocolate is almost melted. Remove pan from heat; continue whisking until chocolate is melted and mixture is smooth. Whisk in egg yolk and vanilla; add Equal®, whisking until smooth.

Beat egg whites and cream of tartar to stiff peaks in large bowl. Fold chocolate mixture into egg whites; fold in combined flour and salt.

Pour cake batter into pan. Bake in preheated 350°F oven until cake is just firm when lightly touched, 18 to 20 minutes, and toothpick inserted in center comes out clean (do not overbake).

Carefully loosen side of cake from pan with small sharp knife to prevent cake from cracking as it cools. Cool cake completely in pan on wire rack; refrigerate until chilled, 1 to 2 hours.

Remove cake from pan and place on serving plate. Spread with Rich Chocolate Glaze, if desired. Garnish with light whipped topping, chocolate drizzle and/or raspberries, if desired.

Nutrients per serving:
Calories: 145, Calories from Fat: 65%, Total Fat: 11g, Saturated Fat: 4g, Cholesterol: 18mg, Sodium: 110mg, Carbohydrate: 11g, Fiber: 2g, Protein: 3g

Dietary Exchanges: 1 Starch, 2 Fat

continued on page 84

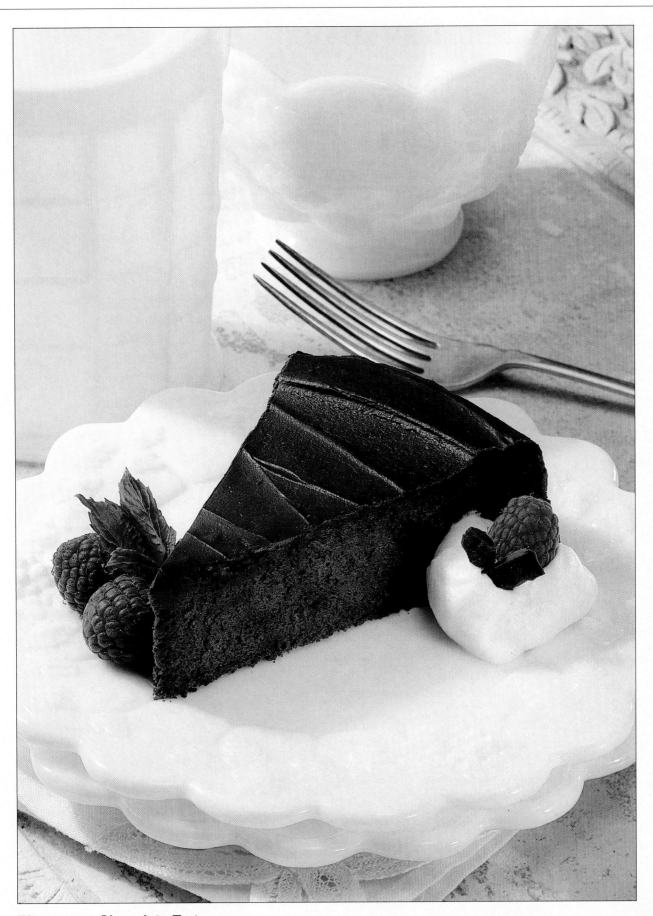

Bittersweet Chocolate Torte

Bittersweet Chocolate Torte, continued

Rich Chocolate Glaze

Makes about ⅓ cup

¼ cup skim milk
2 ounces unsweetened chocolate, cut into small pieces
3½ teaspoons EQUAL® FOR RECIPES *or* 12 packets EQUAL®
sweetener *or* ½ cup EQUAL® SPOONFUL™

Heat milk and chocolate in small saucepan, whisking frequently, until almost melted; remove from heat and whisk until smooth. Whisk in Equal®. Cool to room temperature; refrigerate until thickened enough to spread.

Nutrients per serving: 1/12 of torte + 2 teaspoons glaze
Calories: 175, Calories from Fat: 72%, Total Fat: 14g, Saturated Fat: 4g, Cholesterol: 18mg, Sodium: 113mg, Carbohydrate: 14g, Fiber: 2g, Protein: 4g

Dietary Exchanges: ½ Starch, 2½ Fat

Old-Fashioned Bread Pudding

Makes 12 servings

2 cups fat-free (skim) milk
4 egg whites
3 tablespoons sugar
2 tablespoons margarine, melted
1 tablespoon vanilla
2 teaspoons ground cinnamon
12 slices whole-wheat bread, cut into ½-inch cubes
½ cup raisins
½ cup chopped dried apples

Preheat oven to 350°F. Spray 2-quart casserole with nonstick cooking spray; set aside. Combine milk, egg whites, sugar, margarine, vanilla and cinnamon in large bowl; mix well. Add bread, raisins and dried apples. Allow to stand 5 minutes.

Pour mixture into prepared casserole dish. Bake 35 minutes or until well browned. Cool in pan on wire rack.

Nutrients per serving:
Calories: 150, Calories from Fat: 19%, Total Fat: 3g, Saturated Fat: 1g, Cholesterol: 1mg, Sodium: 214mg, Carbohydrate: 26g, Fiber: 1g, Protein: 6g

Dietary Exchanges: 1 Starch, ½ Fruit, ½ Fat

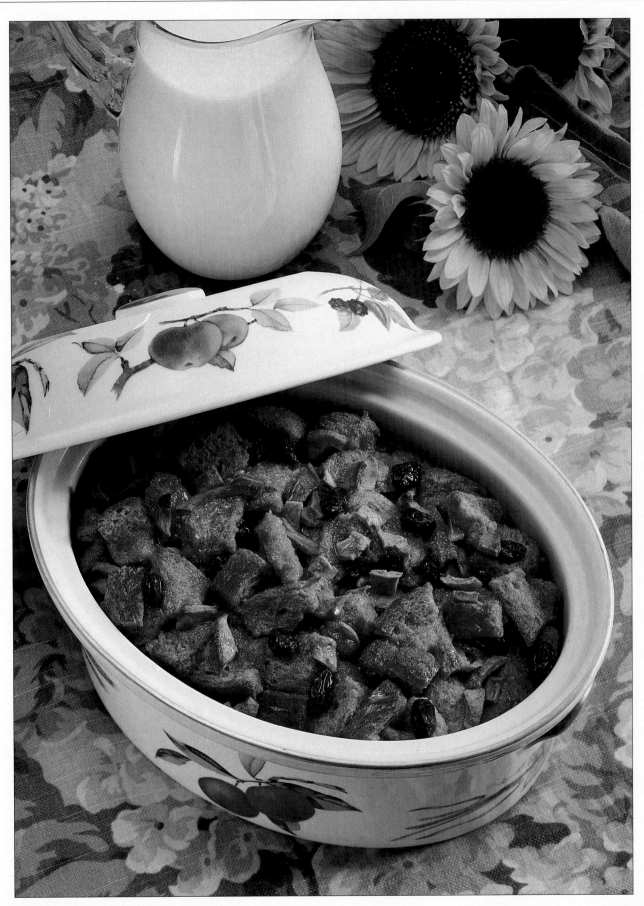

Old-Fashioned Bread Pudding

Lemon Raspberry Tiramisu

Makes 12 servings

>   2 packages (8 ounces each) fat-free cream cheese, softened
>   6 packages sugar substitute *or* equivalent of ¼ cup sugar
>   1 teaspoon vanilla
>   ⅓ cup water
>   1 package (0.3 ounce) sugar-free lemon-flavored gelatin
>   2 cups thawed frozen fat-free nondairy whipped topping
>   ½ cup all-fruit red raspberry preserves
>   ¼ cup water
>   2 tablespoons marsala wine
>   2 packages (3 ounces each) ladyfingers
>   1 pint fresh raspberries or frozen unsweetened raspberries, thawed

Combine cream cheese, sugar substitute and vanilla in large bowl. Beat with electric mixer at high speed until smooth; set aside.

Combine water and gelatin in small microwavable bowl; microwave at HIGH 30 seconds to 1 minute or until water is boiling and gelatin is dissolved. Cool slightly.

Add gelatin mixture to cheese mixture; beat 1 minute. Add whipped topping; beat 1 minute more, scraping side of bowl. Set aside.

Whisk together preserves, water and marsala in small bowl until well blended. Reserve 2 tablespoons of preserves mixture; set aside. Spread ⅓ cup preserves mixture evenly over bottom of 11×7-inch glass baking dish.

Split ladyfingers in half; place half in bottom of baking dish. Spread half of cheese mixture evenly over ladyfingers; sprinkle 1 cup raspberries evenly over cheese mixture. Top with remaining ladyfingers; spread remaining preserves mixture over ladyfingers. Top with remaining cheese mixture. Cover; refrigerate at least 2 hours. Drizzle with reserved 2 tablespoons preserves mixture, and sprinkle with remaining raspberries before serving. Garnish as desired.

Nutrients per serving: ¹⁄₁₂ of recipe
Calories: 158, Calories from Fat: 9%, Total Fat: 1g, Saturated Fat: <1g, Cholesterol: 52mg, Sodium: 272mg, Carbohydrate: 26g, Fiber: 1g, Protein: 7g

Dietary Exchanges: 2 Starch

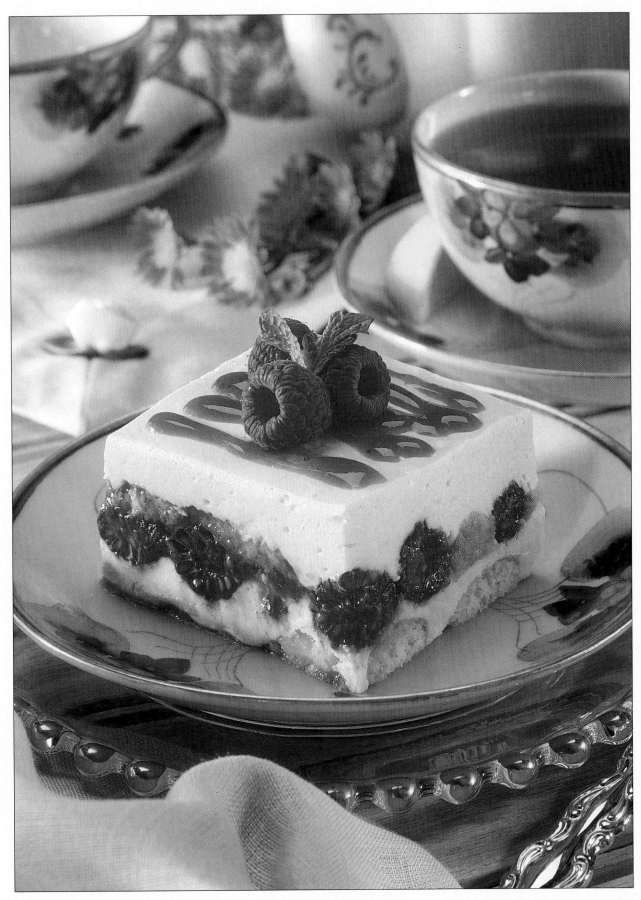

Lemon Raspberry Tiramisu

Double Chocolate Bread Pudding

Makes 12 servings

Prep Time: 15 minutes
Bake Time: 40 minutes plus standing

- **2 packages (4-serving size each) JELL-O® Chocolate Flavor Sugar Free Cook and Serve Pudding & Pie Filling**
- **5 cups fat free milk**
- **5 cups French bread cubes**
- **1 package (4 ounces) BAKER'S® GERMAN'S® Sweet Chocolate, chopped**

HEAT oven to 350°F.

STIR pudding mixes into milk with wire whisk in large bowl 1 minute or until well blended. Stir in bread. Pour pudding mixture into 13×9-inch baking dish. Sprinkle evenly with chopped chocolate.

BAKE 40 minutes or until pudding just comes to a boil in the center. Remove from oven. Let stand 10 minutes before serving. Serve warm. Store leftover pudding in refrigerator.

How to make individual servings: Make individual servings of bread pudding by baking in custard cups or ramekins. Reduce baking time to 15 to 20 minutes. Garnish with COOL WHIP LITE® or COOL WHIP FREE® Whipped Topping.

Dalmatian Bread Pudding: Substitute JELL-O® Vanilla Flavor Sugar Free Cook and Serve Pudding & Pie Filling for Chocolate Flavor Pudding to create a delicious black and white bread pudding.

Nutrients per serving: 1/12 of recipe
Calories: 150, Calories from Fat: 24%, Total Fat: 4g, Saturated Fat: 2g, Cholesterol: <5mg, Sodium: 230mg, Carbohydrate: 26g, Fiber: 2g, Protein: 6g

Dietary Exchanges: 2 Starch, 1/2 Milk

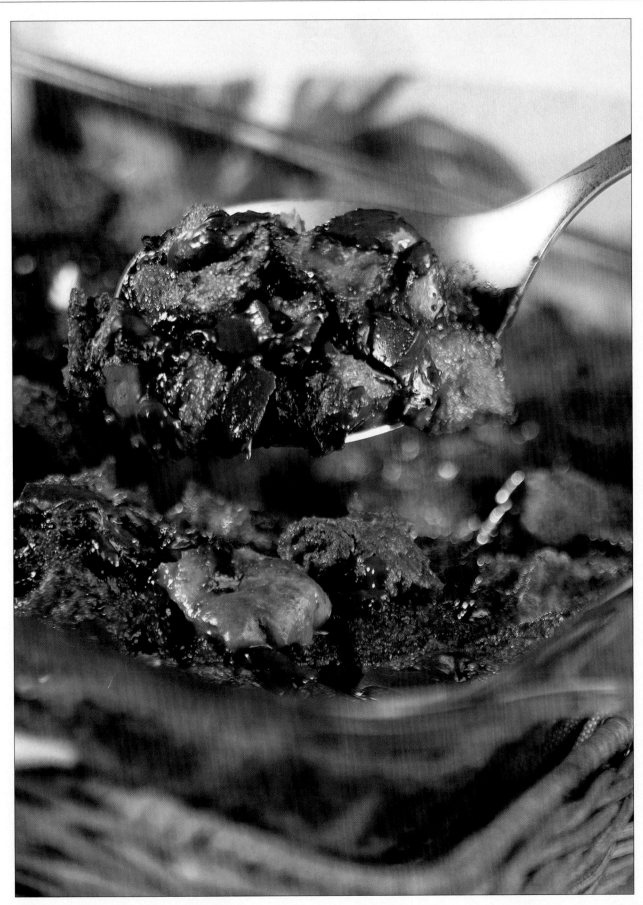

Double Chocolate Bread Pudding

Apple Cranberry Mold

Makes 8 (½-cup) servings

Prep Time: 10 minutes plus refrigerating

> **2 cups boiling apple juice**
> **1 package (8-serving size)** *or* **2 packages (4-serving size each) JELL-O® Brand Cranberry Flavor Sugar Free Low Calorie Gelatin,** *or* **any red flavor**
> **1½ cups reduced calorie cranberry juice cocktail**

STIR boiling juice into gelatin in large bowl at least 2 minutes until completely dissolved. Stir in cranberry juice. Pour into 4-cup mold.

REFRIGERATE 4 hours or until firm. Unmold. Store leftover gelatin mold in refrigerator.

How to Unmold: Dip mold in warm water for about 15 seconds. Gently pull gelatin from around edges with moist fingers. Place moistened serving plate on top of mold. Invert mold and plate; holding mold and plate together, shake slightly to loosen. Gently remove mold and center gelatin on plate.

Nutrients per serving: ½ cup
Calories: 45, Calories from Fat: 0%, Total Fat: 0g, Saturated Fat: 0g, Cholesterol: 0mg, Sodium: 80mg, Carbohydrate: 10g, Fiber: 0g, Protein: 1g

Dietary Exchanges: ½ Fruit

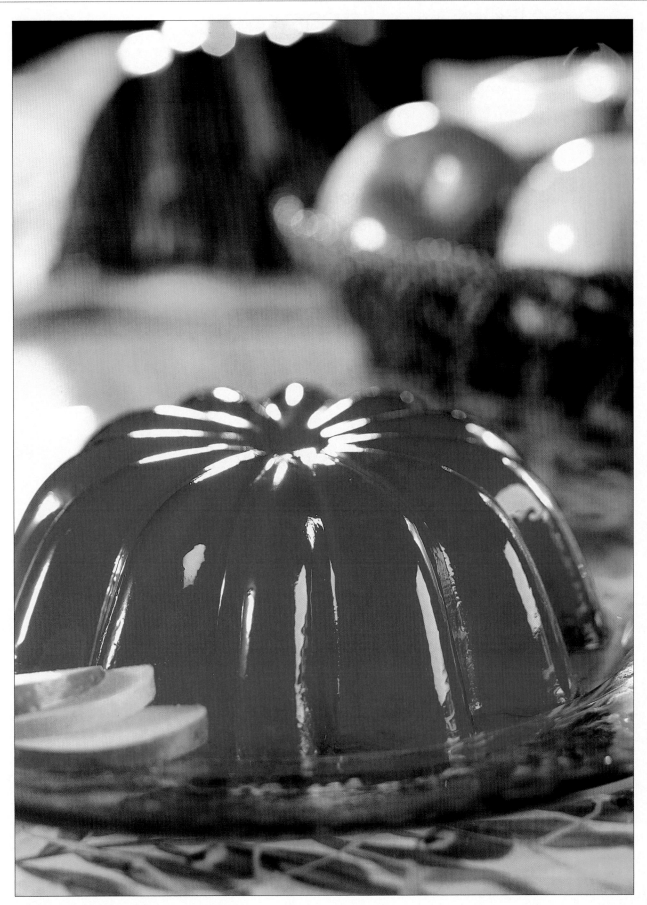

Apple Cranberry Mold

acknowledgments

The publisher would like to thank the companies and organizations listed below for the use of their recipes and photographs in this publication.

Equal® sweetener

Hershey Foods Corporation

Kraft Foods Holdings

index

METRIC CONVERSION CHART

VOLUME MEASUREMENTS (dry)

1/8 teaspoon = 0.5 mL
1/4 teaspoon = 1 mL
1/2 teaspoon = 2 mL
3/4 teaspoon = 4 mL
1 teaspoon = 5 mL
1 tablespoon = 15 mL
2 tablespoons = 30 mL
1/4 cup = 60 mL
1/3 cup = 75 mL
1/2 cup = 125 mL
2/3 cup = 150 mL
3/4 cup = 175 mL
1 cup = 250 mL
2 cups = 1 pint = 500 mL
3 cups = 750 mL
4 cups = 1 quart = 1 L

VOLUME MEASUREMENTS (fluid)

1 fluid ounce (2 tablespoons) = 30 mL
4 fluid ounces (1/2 cup) = 125 mL
8 fluid ounces (1 cup) = 250 mL
12 fluid ounces (1 1/2 cups) = 375 mL
16 fluid ounces (2 cups) = 500 mL

WEIGHTS (mass)

1/2 ounce = 15 g
1 ounce = 30 g
3 ounces = 90 g
4 ounces = 120 g
8 ounces = 225 g
10 ounces = 285 g
12 ounces = 360 g
16 ounces = 1 pound = 450 g

DIMENSIONS

1/16 inch = 2 mm
1/8 inch = 3 mm
1/4 inch = 6 mm
1/2 inch = 1.5 cm
3/4 inch = 2 cm
1 inch = 2.5 cm

OVEN TEMPERATURES

250°F = 120°C
275°F = 140°C
300°F = 150°C
325°F = 160°C
350°F = 180°C
375°F = 190°C
400°F = 200°C
425°F = 220°C
450°F = 230°C

BAKING PAN SIZES

Utensil	Size in Inches/Quarts	Metric Volume	Size in Centimeters
Baking or	8×8×2	2 L	20×20×5
Cake Pan	9×9×2	2.5 L	23×23×5
(square or	12×8×2	3 L	30×20×5
rectangular)	13×9×2	3.5 L	33×23×5
Loaf Pan	8×4×3	1.5 L	20×10×7
	9×5×3	2 L	23×13×7
Round Layer	8×1½	1.2 L	20×4
Cake Pan	9×1½	1.5 L	23×4
Pie Plate	8×1¼	750 mL	20×3
	9×1¼	1 L	23×3
Baking Dish	1 quart	1 L	—
or Casserole	1½ quart	1.5 L	—
	2 quart	2 L	—